Frank A. Chervenak and Laurence B. McCullough

The Professional Responsibility Model of Perinatal Ethics

Hot Topics in Perinatal Medicine

Edited by
Joachim W. Dudenhausen

Volume 2

Frank A. Chervenak and
Laurence B. McCullough

The Professional Responsibility Model of Perinatal Ethics

DE GRUYTER

Frank A. Chervenak, M.D.
New York Weill Cornell Medical Center
Maternal-Fetal Medicine
525 East 68th Street
New York NY 10065
United States of America

Laurence B. McCullough, Ph. D.
Baylor College of Medicine
Center for Medical Ethics & Health Policy
One Baylor Plaza
Houston TX 77030-3411
United States of America

The book has 6 tables.

ISBN 978-3-11-031660-5
e-ISBN 978-3-11-031672-8

Library of Congress Cataloging-in-Publication Data
A CIP catalog record for this book has been applied for at the Library of Congress.

Bibliographic information published by the Deutsche Nationalbibliothek
The Deutsche Nationalbibliothek lists this publication in the Deutsche Nationalbibliografie; detailed bibliographic data are available on the Internet at http://dnb.dnb.de.

Cover image: Comstock/Getty Images
Typesetting: Meta Systems Publishing & Printservices GmbH, Wustermark
Printing and binding: CPI books GmbH, Leck
♾ Printed on acid-free paper
Printed in Germany

www.degruyter.com

This book is for
Drs. Judith Chervenak and Linda J. Quintanilla
for their indefatigable support and tolerance during our more than three decades of collaboration in perinatal ethics

Preface

When the authors started their collaboration in perinatal ethics in 1983, ethics was often relegated to the fringes of perinatal practice, research, and education. Today, perinatologists have awakened to the essential role of ethics in elucidating professional responsibility in their specialty. This is why we have entitled this book, *The Professional Responsibility Model of Perinatal Ethics.*

The book has ten chapters that cover the spectrum of clinical and research challenges faced by perinatologists on a day-to-day basis. The first chapter provides an ethical framework based on the two core concepts of the professional responsibility model of perinatal ethics, the ethical concepts of medicine as a profession and of the pregnant woman, fetus and neonate as patients. We present the professional responsibility model as an antidote to fetal rights-based reductionist and maternal rights-based reductionist approaches that result in gridlock and undermine professionalism in perinatology. Rooted in the medical ethics of the Scottish and English Enlightenments of the eighteenth century, the professional responsibility model is secular and therefore transreligious, transcultural, and transnational. The professional responsibility model is distinctive in its emphasis on a preventive ethics approach to the ethical challenges of perinatology.

The subsequent chapters address ethical challenges in clinical practice (Chapters 2–7) and innovation and research (Chapter 8). Advocacy for the health and healthcare of women and children is a major component of professional responsibility in perinatology and is therefore addressed in Chapter 9. Lastly, perinatal ethics is not mere opinion, but an intellectually and clinically disciplined approach to the identification, prevention, and management of ethical challenges in perinatology. In Chapter 10, we therefore provide the reader with a tool for the critical appraisal of the literature of perinatal ethics.

The authors are convinced that, in the more than three decades since we began our work, ethics has become an indefeasible part of perinatal medicine that defines the professional perinatologist.

Frank A. Chervenak,
Laurence B. McCullough

Contents

1 The professional responsibility model of perinatal ethics

1.1 Introduction

Perinatologists confront an impressive range of ethical challenges in clinical practice and in research designed to benefit maternal and fetal patients. The responsible management of these ethical challenges, therefore, becomes essential to the professional practice of perinatology and to perinatal research. The purpose of this book is to introduce the reader to the two basic tools of ethics – ethical analysis and ethical argument – and to demonstrate how these two tools of ethics generate a practical, clinically comprehensive, professional medical ethics for perinatal practice and research.

Throughout the chapters that follow, we emphasize a preventive ethics approach.[1,2] Preventive ethics aims to prevent ethical conflict in clinical practice by anticipating the potential for ethical conflict and designing ethically justified, practical approaches designed to minimize the occurrence of ethical conflict and to respond rapidly and effectively to ethical conflicts when, despite sustained effort to prevent them, they nonetheless occur.

The methodological basis for the approach to perinatal ethics taken in this book is the professional responsibility model of perinatal ethics. In this chapter, we introduce this model, after first providing definitions of ethics, medical ethics, and perinatal ethics.

1.2 Ethics, medical ethics, and perinatal ethics

1.2.1 Ethics

Ethics has been understood for millennia in global intellectual, cultural, and religious traditions to constitute the disciplined study of morality. Morality concerns our beliefs about what sort of people we should aspire to become; our obligations to each other, to our communities, to organizations, and society; the obligations of organizations to individuals, communities, and society; and the obligations of society to individuals, communities, and organizations. Ethics seeks to identify and critically assess those beliefs, with the goal of improving morality.

Ethics undertakes this task by asking, What ought morality to be? To make this question more manageable and to generate practical answers that will guide the improvement of morality, this general question is broken down into specific questions: What sort of persons should we become? How should we act toward each other, communities, organizations, and society? How should organizations act toward each other, individuals, communities, and society? How should society act toward individuals, communities, and organizations?

The tools of ethical reasoning. These questions are addressed using the two basic tools of ethics; ethical analysis and argument. Ethical analysis requires us to be clear about concepts, such as being a patient and professional integrity, that we invoke and to use those concepts with a consistent meaning to give reasons for our judgments and behavior based on them. Ethical argument requires us to join ethical concepts together in a coherent way to provide reasons that together support conclusions. Simply listing disconnected ethical considerations does not count as argument. Neither does starting with conclusions, and then going in search of supportive ethical considerations.

The discipline of ethics comes from two sources. The first relates to ethical analysis: adhering to the requirements of clarity and consistency in the articulation of ethical concepts. The second relates to ethical argument: identifying the implications of clearly articulated, ethical concepts for clinical practice and research, or going where our arguments take us and nowhere else. The discipline of ethical argument has an important feature: If one is not willing to accept the conclusion of an argument, one must show an error in the reasoning that supports it, correct the error, and then identify the revised or even new conclusion that follows from the revised reasons. If one cannot do so, then one is required to change one's mind by adopting the conclusion. This discipline of ethical argument is directly analogous to the discipline of deliberative (evidence-based, rigorous, transparent, and accountable) clinical judgment: When the evidence requires one to change one's clinical judgment, the professionally responsible physician does so. The professionally responsible physician, by submitting to the disciplined study of morality that is ethics, sometimes will be required to change his or her clinical ethical judgment.

1.2.2 Medical ethics

Medical ethics is the disciplined study of morality in medicine. Medical ethics undertakes this study by asking specific questions: What does it mean to say that a physician is a professional? What obligations do physicians owe their patients, healthcare organizations, and society? What obligations do patients owe their physicians, healthcare organizations, and society? What obligations do healthcare organizations owe their patients, healthcare professionals, and society? What obligations do societies have to physicians, patients, and healthcare organizations?

Medical ethics should not be confused with the many sources of morality in a pluralistic society. These include, but are not limited to, law, the world's religions, ethnic and cultural traditions, families, and personal experience. Professional medical ethics seeks to bridge these differences and identify the obligations of physicians to their patients in all global cultures, religions, and national settings.

Medical ethics as secular. The first step in doing so is to recognize that professional medical ethics is secular. This recognition was achieved in the eighteenth-century European and American Enlightenments.[4] Secular professional medical ethics makes no reference to deity or deities, or to revealed tradition, but to what reasoned, evidence-based discourse requires of our judgments and behavior. At the same time, secular professional medical ethics is not intrinsically hostile to but respectful of religious beliefs. Therefore, ethical principles and virtues should be understood to apply to all physicians, regardless of their personal religious and spiritual beliefs, and regardless of their nationality or place of practice.[5] The advantage of secular medical ethics is that it is transreligious, transcultural, and transnational.[3]

The traditions and practices of medicine constitute an obvious source of morality for physicians. These traditions provide an important reference point for professional medical ethics because they are based on the obligation to protect and promote the health-related interests of the patient. This obligation tells physicians what morality in medicine ought to be, but only in very general, abstract terms. Providing a clinically applicable account of that obligation is, in clinical practice, the central task of professional medical ethics, using ethical principles.[2,5] We start with ethical principles that play a central role in professional medical ethics; beneficence and respect for autonomy. The ethical principle of justice will be introduced in Chapter 2, and more extensively in Chapter 3.

The ethical principle of beneficence. In ethics, generally, the ethical principle of beneficence requires one to act in a way that is reliably expected to produce a greater balance of benefits over harms in the lives of others.[2,5] In professional medical ethics, this principle requires the physician to seek a greater balance of clinical gods over clinical harms in the lives of patients.[2] The task of beneficence-based clinical judgment is to reach reasoned judgments about the appropriate balance of clinical goods and harms in a particular clinical situation, such as the decision to perform a cesarean delivery (see Chapter 4).

Beneficence-based clinical judgment has an ancient pedigree. Its first expression in the history of Western medical ethics occurs in the Hippocratic Oath and accompanying texts.[6] These texts make an important claim: to reliably interpret the health related interests of the patient from a deliberative clinical perspective. This perspective is provided by accumulated scientific research, clinical experience, and reasoned responses to uncertainty. A rigorously evidence-based, beneficence-based clinical judgment is not based on the idiosyncratic judgment of the physician, i.e. merely on the clinical impression or intuition of an individual physician. On the basis of this deliberative clinical perspective, focused on the best available evidence, beneficence-based clinical judgment identifies the clinical benefits that can be achieved for the patient by the clinical application of the competencies of medicine. These competencies are the prevention and management of disease, injury, disability, loss of functional status, and unnecessary pain, distress, and suffering, and the prevention of premature or unnecessary death. Pain and suffering become unnecessary when they do not result in achieving the other goods of clinical care, e.g. allowing a woman to labor without effective analgesia.[2]

In beneficence-based clinical judgment, pregnancy is not a disease. It is, instead, a clinical condition: a naturally occurring biological process that creates risks of disease, injury, disability, loss of functional status, and unnecessary pain, distress, and suffering. As a consequence, the clinical management of the clinical condition of pregnancy comes under beneficence-based clinical judgment.

The ethical principle of non-maleficence. The ethical principle of non-maleficence requires the physician not to cause harm. This is sometimes treated as an absolute, allowing no exceptions. This is a common mistake; non-maleficence is best understood as expressing the limits of beneficence-based clinical judgment. This ethical principle is also known as *Primum non nocere* or "first do no harm." This commonly invoked dogma is really a latinized misinterpretation of the Hippocratic texts, which emphasized beneficence while avoiding harm when approaching the limits of the competencies of medicine, especially to maintain or improve the patient's condition, or to alter the course of disease or injury.[2,5] The Ancient Greek physicians got it right: non-maleficence should be subsumed under beneficence-based clinical judgment.

We emphasize that there is an inherent risk of paternalism (interfering with a patient's autonomy for the patient's good) in beneficence-based clinical judgment. By this we mean that beneficence-based clinical judgment, if it is *mistakenly* considered to be the sole source, not just of professional responsibility but also of moral authority to control the course of obstetric care, invites the unwary perinatologist to conclude that beneficence-based judgments can simply be imposed on the pregnant woman in violation of her autonomy. Paternalism dehumanizes the treatment of the pregnant woman and, therefore, should be avoided in obstetric practice.

The ethical principle of respect for autonomy. The antidote to paternalism is respect for the pregnant woman's autonomy.[2,5] This ethical principle requires the physician to empower the pregnant woman to make informed, deliberative, and voluntary (free of controlling external and internal influences[7]) decisions about the management of her pregnancy. The most important way that physicians fulfill this obligation is to identify medically reasonable alternatives to the pregnant woman and to identify alternatives that, while technically possible, are reliably judged to be not medically reasonable. "Medically reasonable" means that there is a beneficence-based clinical judgment that a form of clinical management or intervention has a reliable evidence base for expected net clinical benefit. There is no ethical obligation to offer a technically possible alternative that does not meet this test for being medically reasonable.

The informed consent process. When the condition for being medically reasonable is met, the alternative should be offered, along with the other medically reasonable alternatives. Sometimes the evidence clearly supports one alternative as clinically superior to others or as the only medically reasonable alternative. In such clinical circumstances, the physician should recommend this alternative to the pregnant woman. Sometimes the evidence clearly rules out an alternative as not medically reasonable, or medically unreasonable. In such clinical circumstances, the physician should not offer this alternative to the pregnant woman and should recommend against it should the pregnant woman ask about it.

Patients' decision-making capacity. Patients exercise their capacity for autonomous decision making in response to alternatives that are offered or recommended by the physician in the informed consent process. The capacity for autonomous decision making has three components. 1) absorbing and retaining information about her condition and the medically reasonable diagnostic and therapeutic responses to it; 2) understanding that information, i.e. evaluating and rank-ordering those responses and appreciating that she could experience the risks of treatment; and 3) expressing a value-based preference.[8] The physician has a role to play in each of these. They are, respectively: 1) to recognize the capacity of each patient to deal with medical information and not to underestimate that capacity, provide information (i.e. disclose and explain all medically reasonable alternatives) and recognize the validity of the values and beliefs of the patient; 2) not to interfere with but, when necessary, to assist the patient in her evaluation and ranking of the medically reasonable diagnostic and therapeutic alternatives for managing her condition; and 3) to elicit and implement the patient's value-based preference.[2]

United States common law on simple and informed consent. The common law in the United States played an important role in clarifying the physician's obligation to provide information to the patient, to empower her to make informed decisions. The common law made the important contribution of identifying the concept of simple consent. The concept of simple consent was established in a landmark gynecologic case, *Schloendorff v. The Society of The New York Hospital.* Simple consent concerns whether the patient says "yes" or "no" to medical intervention.[7,9] To this day in the medical and bioethics literature, this decision is quoted: "Every human being of adult years and sound mind has the right to determine what shall be done with his body, and a surgeon who performs an operation without his patient's consent commits an assault for which he is liable in damages."[9]

The concept of informed consent further evolved in the common law to include disclosure of information sufficient to enable patients to make informed decisions about whether to say "yes" or "no" to medical intervention.[7] Two accepted legal standards emerged: the professional community standard; and the reasonable person standard.

The professional community standard defines adequate disclosure in the context of what relevantly trained and experienced physicians actually tell their patients. The reasonable person standard, which has been adopted by most states in the United States (where the states regulate the practice of medicine, not the federal government), goes further and requires the physician to disclose "material" information. This phase means information that any patient in a particular patient's condition needs to know and that the lay person of average sophistication should not be expected to know. This is a very abstract formulation of the concept of material information. It can be made clinically applicable in a straightforward way: Patients need to know what the physician thinks is clinically salient, i.e. the physician's beneficence-based clinical judgment about medically reasonable alternatives: what they involve and their clinical benefits and risks.

The reasonable person standard has emerged as the accepted ethical standard.[2,7] We therefore adopt it in this book. On this standard, the physician should disclose to the pregnant patient her or the fetus's diagnosis (including differential diagnosis when that is all that is known), the medically reasonable alternatives to diagnose and manage the patient's condition, the short-term and long-term clinical benefits and risks of each alternative, and the evidence-based, deliberative clinical ethical judgment of the physician that the clinical benefits outweigh the clinical harms. When in deliberative clinical judgment, there is only one medically reasonable alternative, or when one is clinically superior to others in its outcomes, it should be recommended.

Patients' preferences. Respect for autonomy does not require the physician to implement a patient's preference simply on the basis that the patient has freely expressed it. Put another way, the exercise of rights by the patient should not be regarded as an absolute determinant of the physician's clinical practice.[2,10,11]

1.2.3 Perinatal ethics

Perinatal ethics is the disciplined study of morality in perinatal medicine. Perinatal ethics undertakes this study by asking: What does it mean to say that the perinatologist is a professional? What obligations do perinatologists owe to pregnant, fetal, and neonatal patients? What obligations do pregnant women owe to the fetal and neonatal patient, physicians, healthcare organizations, and society? What obligations do healthcare organizations owe to pregnant, fetal, and neonatal patients, physicians, and society? What obligations does society owe to pregnant, fetal, and neonatal patients, physicians, and healthcare organizations?

Ethical obligations to pregnant and fetal patients. The ethical principles of beneficence and respect for autonomy should guide professional perinatal clinical judgment and practice. There are beneficence-based and autonomy-based obligations to the pregnant patient. The perinatologist's perspective on the pregnant woman's health-related interests provides the basis for the perinatologist's beneficence-based obligations to her, whereas her own perspective on those interests provides the basis for the perinatologist's autonomy-based obligations to her, as described above. Because of an insufficiently developed central nervous system, the fetus cannot meaningfully be said to possess values and beliefs. Thus, there is no basis for saying that a fetus has a perspective on its interests. There can, therefore, be no autonomy-based obligations to any fetus.

The fetus as a patient. Obviously, the perinatologist has a perspective on the fetus's health-related interests, and the physician can therefore have beneficence-based obligations to the fetus, *but only when the fetus is a patient*. Because of its importance for obstetric clinical judgment and practice, the ethical concept of the fetus as a patient requires detailed consideration.[2]

Developments in fetal diagnosis and management strategies to optimize fetal outcome have become widely accepted, encouraging the development of the ethical concept of the fetus as a patient. This concept has considerable clinical significance because, when the fetus is a patient, directive counseling, that is, recommending a form of management for fetal benefit is appropriate. When the fetus is not a patient, nondirective counseling, that is, offering but not recommending a form of management for fetal benefit is appropriate.[2]

One prominent approach for establishing whether or not the fetus is a patient attempts to show whether or not the fetus has independent moral status. The ethical concept of independent moral status for the fetus means that one or more characteristics that the fetus possesses in and of itself, and therefore independently of the pregnant woman, the perinatologist or society, generate and therefore ground obligations to the fetus on the part of the pregnant woman and her physician. Many fetal characteristics have been nominated for this role, including moment of conception, implantation, central nervous system development, quickening, and the moment of birth.[12] It should come as no surprise that there is considerable variation among ethical arguments about when the fetus acquires independent moral status. One view is that the fetus has independent moral status from the moment of conception or implantation.[12] Another view is that independent moral status is acquired in degrees, thus resulting in "graded" moral status.[13] Still another view holds, at least by implication, that the fetus never has independent moral status so long as it is *in utero*.[14]

Despite a centuries-old global, and an ever-expanding theological and philosophical literature on this subject, there has been no closure on a single authoritative account of the independent moral status of the fetus. Given the absence of a single method that would be authoritative for all of the markedly diverse theological and philosophical schools of thought involved in this very long debate, closure is impossible and therefore should not be expected. Readers should be very skeptical of claims that a single account of the independent moral status of the fetus is universally authoritative. All attempts to explain the ethical concept on the basis of the purported independent moral status of the fetus are irresolvably controversial, and thus provide no reliable clinical basis for the clarification or clinical application of the concept.

A clinically reliable explanation of the ethical concept of the fetus as a patient starts with the recognition that being a patient does not require that one possess independent moral status.[15] The ethical concept of being a patient is clinically straightforward: a human being (1) is presented to a physician (or other healthcare professional such as a nurse midwife) and (2) there exist clinical interventions that are reliably expected to be clinically effective: they are reliably expected to result in a greater balance of clinical benefits over harms for the human being in question. In the technical language of ethics, generally, this is known as the dependent moral status of the fetus.[2]

The authors have argued elsewhere that beneficence-based obligations to the fetus exist when the fetus is reliably expected *later* to achieve dependent moral status as a child and then independent moral status as a person.[2] That is, the fetus is a patient when the fetus is presented for medical interventions, whether diagnostic or therapeutic, that reasonably can be expected to result in a greater balance of goods over harms for the fetus, and therefore for the child and person the fetus can *later* become during early childhood. The ethical significance of the concept of the fetus as a patient, therefore, depends on links that can be established between the fetus and its later achieving independent moral status.

The viable fetal patient. One such link is viability, the ability of the fetus to exist ex utero, albeit with full technological support. Viability, however, must be understood in terms of *both* biological and technological factors. It is only by virtue of *both factors* that a viable fetus can exist ex utero, and thus achieve independent moral status. When a fetus is viable, that is, when it is of sufficient maturity so that it can survive into the neonatal period and achieve independent moral status given the availability of the requisite technological support, and when it is presented to the physician, the fetus is a patient.

Viability exists as a function of biomedical and technological capacities, which are different in different parts of the world. As a consequence, there is, at the present time, no worldwide, uniform gestational age to define viability. In the United States, we believe, viability presently occurs at approximately 24 weeks of gestational age.[16,17] (See Chapter 3)

The previable fetal patient. Before viability, the only link between the fetus and its later becoming a child is the pregnant woman's decision to continue her pregnancy to viability. The previable fetus is, therefore, a patient solely as a function of the pregnant woman's autonomous decision to confer this moral status on her fetus(es).[2] Prior to viability, none of the interventions of perinatal medicine can benefit the fetus without the pregnant woman's body as the necessary condition for later becoming a child and person. After viability, there is much that perinatal medicine can do to benefit the fetus, which, because it can exist ex utero (even with full technological support), no longer needs the pregnant woman's body as a necessary condition for later becoming a child and person. Neither before nor after viability, however, should the fetus be considered a separate patient, i.e. the beneficence-based obligations to whom are all that need to be considered. Deliberative clinical ethical judgment about professional responsibility to the fetus as a patient always requires taking into account not only beneficence-based obligations to the fetus, but also beneficence-based and autonomy-based obligations to the pregnant woman.

Directive counseling for fetal benefit. When the fetus is a patient, directive counseling for fetal benefit is ethically justified. In clinical practice, directive counseling for fetal benefit involves one or more of the following: recommending against termination of pregnancy; recommending against nonaggressive management; or recommending aggressive management. Aggressive obstetric management includes interventions such as fetal surveillance, tocolysis, cesarean delivery, or delivery in a tertiary care center when indicated. Nonaggressive obstetric management excludes such interventions. Directive counseling for fetal benefit, however, must take account of the presence and severity of fetal anomalies, extreme prematurity, and obligations to the pregnant woman.

Directive counseling for fetal benefit must occur in the context of balancing beneficence-based obligations to the fetus against beneficence-based and autonomy-based obligations to the pregnant woman. Such balancing must recognize that a pregnant woman is obligated only to take reasonable risks of medical interventions that are reliably expected to benefit the fetal and neonatal patient.[2]

The neonatal patient. When the fetus is born alive, the fetal patient becomes a neonatal patient. Perinatal ethics for the neonatal patient is guided by the core ethical concept of pediatric ethics, the best interests of the child standard.[18] The best interests of the child standard generates the ethical obligations of perinatologists and parents to the child, who is a patient.

Decision-making authority of perinatologists and parents. Because deliberative clinical judgment requires clinical expertise, the reliability of the perinatologist's deliberative clinical judgment about biomedical best interests of the child will, as a rule, be greater than the reliability of the parent's clinical judgment about the biomedical best interests of the child. The degree or strength of the reliability of the perinatologist's deliberative clinical judgment, in all cases, is a function of the level and quality of its evidence base. The stronger the evidence base, the stronger the reliability of the perinatologist's deliberative judgment about the biomedical bests interests of the child. When the evidence base is strong, the perinatologist should be directive in not only offering medically reasonable alternatives but recommending the medically reasonable alternative. The weaker the evidence base, the weaker the reliability of the perinatologist's deliberative clinical judgment. When the evidence base is weak, the perinatologist should offer but not recommend medically reasonable alternatives. This is especially the case when non-intervention may be as medically reasonable as intervention. Shared decision making becomes the appropriate approach in such cases.

The evidence base for deliberative clinical judgment about the psychological best interests of a pediatric patient is, as a rule, weaker than that for biomedical best interests. In addition, parents often have equal or even greater insight into the psychological well-being of their child. Neither the perinatologist nor the parent can claim sole prerogative to make judgments about the psychological bests interests of the child. The perinatologist should offer and recommend intervention when the evidence base for it is strong. When the evidence base is weak, the perinatologist should offer but not recommend intervention and engage the pregnant woman in shared decision making.

The evidence base for deliberative clinical judgment about the social best interests of the child is, as a rule, weaker than that for the psychological best interests. For example, contact sports are biomedically risky for growing children, but in many countries and cultures there may be a strong social expectation that children should participate in such sports. Indeed, there is often little or no reliable evidence for clinical judgments about the social best interests of the child. As a consequence, the reliability of parental judgment may be equal or even superior to the reliability of the pediatrician's judgment. Shared decision making should therefore be the approach. The perinatologist should offer intervention and explain the limits of its evidence base, elicit the parents' views and judgments, and work toward a consensus clinical judgment about the social best interests of the child.

Quality-of-life (engaging in valued life tasks and deriving satisfaction from doing so) considerations do not apply to neonatal patients, because they are not yet developmentally capable of having life tasks. Quality-of-life considerations also do not apply to children whose neurologic condition precludes having valued life tasks, i.e. children who have irreversibly lost the capacity to interact with the environment, and thus grow and develop. There is also a more general problem with applying the concept of quality of life in neonatal and pediatric ethics. Saigal and Tyson consider self-reported quality of life, its most reliable measure. Their review of the literature on the self-reported quality of life of individuals who are survivors of neonatal care leads them to conclude that "having a biological impairment does not automatically translate into a poor self-assessed quality of life."[19] It follows directly that predictions about future quality of life of neonates with disabling conditions lack support in deliberative clinical judgment, and therefore should not be made. Because there is, therefore, no scientific foundation for predictive judgments of quality of life by physicians or parents, it is ethically impermissible to use the concept of quality of life to make such predictions in perinatal practice.

Parental authority and rights. The best interests of the child standard has an important implication for the ethics of parental authority over their children who are patients. Parental rights of decision making about the healthcare of a pediatric patient are a function of parents fulfilling their beneficence-based obligation to protect and promote the health-related interests of their child. To the extent that parents do not do so, for whatever reason they may have or express, their ethical authority over their child diminishes. Deliberative clinical ethical judgment must take into account whether the interests of child at stake are biomedical, psychological, or social and the strength of the evidence base for each before reaching a judgment that parental authority over a pediatric patient should be limited.

This aspect of perinatal ethics stands in sharp contrast to counseling pregnant women in the informed consent process about the management of pregnancy. Pregnant women have beneficence-based obligations to protect the life and health of the fetal patient but are ethically obligated only to take reasonable risks to themselves to fulfill those obligations.[2] Deliberative clinical ethical judgment must, therefore, always take into account not only the perinatologist's and pregnant woman's beneficence-based obligations to the fetal patient but also the perinatologist's beneficence-based and autonomy-based obligations to the pregnant woman. Delivery makes an ethical difference: Perinatal ethics during pregnancy and perinatal ethics after delivery differ because the ethical obligations to a fetal patient and ethical obligations to a neonatal patient differ significantly. In all cases, beneficence-based obligations to the fetal patient must be balanced against beneficence-based and autonomy-based obligations to the pregnant woman, who is the sole decision maker. For neonatal patients, the perinatologist's obligations to the neonatal patient are beneficence-based and both parents are decision makers but not patients.

1.3 The professional responsibility model of perinatal ethics

The professional responsibility model of perinatal ethics guides perinatologists in responsibly managing ethical challenges in clinical practice and research. In all obstetric decision making, this model requires the perinatologist to identity three sets of ethical obligations: beneficence-based and autonomy-based obligations to the pregnant woman and beneficence-based obligations to the fetal patient. In almost all clinical circumstances these three obligations are congruent; conflicts are rare. Sometimes, however, these three obligations can come into conflict. Conflict between or among these obligations should be managed on the basis of deliberative clinical ethical judgment. For example, directive counseling for fetal benefit must take account of obligations to the pregnant woman, which creates the possibility of conflict between the physician's recommendation and a pregnant woman's autonomous decision to the contrary. Such conflict is best managed preventively through the informed consent process, guided by deliberative clinical ethical judgment, as an ongoing dialogue throughout a woman's pregnancy, augmented as necessary by negotiation and respectful persuasion.[1,2] Respectful persuasion guides the perinatologist to appeal to the pregnant woman's values, such as achieving a good outcome for her pregnancy, make recommendations based on those values, and respond to refusal with engaged dialogue aiming at having the pregnant woman reconsider her refusal. In all neonatal decision making, this model requires the perinatologist to identify which technically possible clinical management protects and promotes the health-related interest of the neonatal patient and is, therefore, medically reasonable. Parents usually authorize such clinical management. Conflict with parents should be guided by deliberative clinical ethical judgment deployed in the informed consent process, followed by negotiation and respectful persuasion as needed.

This approach to perinatal ethics in both obstetric and neonatal practice is known as the professional responsibility model of perinatal ethics and is based on the professional responsibility model of obstetric ethics.[3] The professional responsibility model of perinatal ethics provides a powerful antidote to the rights-based reductionism that characterizes much of the literature on perinatal ethics. This oversimplification of perinatal ethics occurs when the only or overriding ethical consideration is rights of either the pregnant woman or the fetus.

1.3.1 Rights-based reductionism

Right-based reductionism is best illustrated by the abortion controversy. One extreme asserts that fetal rights always override the rights of the pregnant woman. This is fetal-rights reductionism. Termination of pregnancy at any gestational age or for any reason is impermissible, regardless of whether the pregnancy is voluntary or not or viable or not.[20] The other extreme asserts that the pregnant woman's rights always override fetal rights. This is maternal-rights reductionism. Termination of pregnancy is, therefore, permissible at any gestational age and for any reason.[21,22]

Such rights-talk is initially appealing because of the simple dichotomy at its heart: one either has rights or one does not and, if one does, others must respect one's rights. This simple dichotomy is simplistic and does not withstand close clinical ethical scrutiny. There is unavoidable controversy about the nature and limits of both fetal and women's rights. Such rights are based on many factors, including cultural, political, and religious beliefs that do not lend themselves to compromise and are outside of the physician-patient relationship.

Consider the simplistic claim that a pregnant woman has the unconditional right to control what happens to her body. The claim ignores a fundamental question: should this right be understood to come with limits or with no exceptions throughout the entire pregnancy? Professional integrity sets justified limits on the preferences of patients,[10,11] pregnant patients included. For example, a distraught woman who is thirty-four weeks pregnant reports that her husband has deserted her and insists on induced abortion immediately. The professional responsibility model requires her perinatologist not to implement her request because feticide is ruled out by the perinatologist's beneficence-based obligation to protect the life of this fetal patient. The obstetrician should, therefore, recommend against feticide and explain that no conscientious obstetrician should implement her request.

There are many such circumstances in which a pregnant woman's request for an induced abortion should not be implemented unquestioningly.

Consider the simplistic claim that the fetus has an unconditional right to life or to complete gestation. The presence of a fetal anomaly incompatible with life belies such claims as lacking scientific and clinical foundation, because medicine has no capacity to correct such anomalies. Such claims lack an authoritative foundation in either religion or philosophy, because there is no right to the impossible. There is no single authoritative perspective from which the incompatible differences of these diverse views on fetal rights can be resolved.[2] To insist on an unconditional right to life or to complete gestation therefore has no place in professional perinatal ethics.

The existence of maternal-rights reductionism approach in the literature is well documented in the context of an important topic in perinatal ethics, intrapartum management (see Chapter 4). This approach asserts an unconditional right of the pregnant woman to control her body in all aspects of the management of pregnancy: "... the moral and legal primacy of the competent, informed pregnant woman in decision making is overwhelming."[14] Another expression of this approach at first seems to be non-reductionist. Its authors acknowledge patient safety as a "first-order issue"[21] and support what they call "restrictive guidelines" based on protecting the life and health of pregnant women.[21] The proponents of this seemingly nuanced approach, however, abandoned it in favor of the maternal-rights reductionism model when they asserted: "Crucially, even when restrictive guidelines are warranted, the rights of pregnant women to bodily integrity must be maintained."[22] Some express this approach explicitly, e.g. that "women have fully endowed rights that do not diminish with conception, nor progressively degrade as pregnancy advances to viability and birth."[22] The woman's-rights reductionism approach has been used to claim the right of pregnant women to have a clinically non-indicated cesarean delivery.[23,24] Another example is the assertion of the pregnant woman's autonomy as an "unrestricted negative right," i.e. an unconditional right to non-interference with refusal of cesarean delivery: "autonomy is an inter-relational right – ultimately there is no circumstance in which someone should be brought to an operating room against their will."[25]

Rights-based reductionism has no place in perinatal ethics, because it unacceptably distorts the professional nature of the relationship of a perinatologist with his or her patients. The professional obligations of the perinatologist originate in the ethical concept of medicine as a profession.

1.3.2 The ethical concept of medicine as a profession

The concept of medicine as a professional was introduced into the history of medicine by Drs. John Gregory (1724–1773) of Scotland and Thomas Percival (1740–

1804) of England. This concept requires the physician to make three commitments: (1) becoming and remaining scientifically and clinically competent; (2) protecting and promoting the health-related and other interests of the patient as the physician's primary concern and motivation; and (3) preserving and strengthening medicine as what Percival called a "public trust," a social institution that exists primarily for the benefit of society not its members (in contrast to the concept of medicine as a merchant guild, which had dominated in the history of medicine from the time ancient Greece and especially since Medieval and Renaissance Europe).[26]

In the professional responsibility model of perinatal ethics, perinatologists have beneficence-based an autonomy-based obligations to the pregnant patient and beneficence-based obligations to the fetal patient.[2,3] The beneficence-based obligation of the perinatologist is to make evidence-based clinical judgments about diagnostic and therapeutic measures that are reliably expected to result in a greater balance of clinical goods over clinical harms for the pregnant or fetal patient. The perinatologist then empowers the pregnant woman's autonomy by offering or recommending medically reasonable alternatives, as explained above.

The professional responsibility model of perinatal ethics, therefore, includes emphasis on the decision-making rights of the pregnant woman. She has the right to be adequately informed about the medically reasonable alternatives for the management of her pregnancy, and she has the right to authorize such clinical management or refuse it. These rights include the right to elect induced abortion or termination of pregnancy, as we elucidate in Chapter 2. The professional responsibility model is distinctive in that the pregnant woman's rights are sometimes justifiably limited. In the technical language of ethics, the pregnant woman's rights are *prima facie,* not absolute.

The contrast with rights-based reductionism is stark, because it makes the rights of the pregnant woman absolute. Fetal rights-reductionism, despite its simplicity and powerful initial appeal, has no place in perinatal ethics because it inevitably leads perinatal ethics into conceptual and clinical failure. This model, therefore, should be abandoned. Maternal-rights reductionism is a failure as well and requires the perinatologist to implement birth plans that unconditionally exclude cesarean delivery or the unconditional right to planned home birth.[27] Both approaches eliminate the perinatologist's beneficence-based obligations to *both* the pregnant and fetal patients, and therefore reduces the perinatologist to a mere technician, indeed automaton. Maternal-rights reductionism also has absurd implications, e.g. ruling out, as potential paternalism, strongly and repeatedly recommending that pregnant women who abuse tobacco and alcohol seek help and be supported in doing so. Respect for the pregnant woman's rights allows simply accepting such clinically choices by patients because they have made clinically unwise, but autonomous, choices. This is abandonment from the perspective of professional responsibility for patients. Maternal-rights reductionism, despite its simplicity and powerful appeal for many, has no place in perinatal ethics because it inevitably leads perinatal ethics to conceptual and clinical failure. This model, therefore, should also be abandoned.

1.4 Conclusion

The professional responsibility model of perinatal ethics is based on the pioneering medical ethics of two major figures in its history, Drs. John Gregory and Thomas Percival. The ethical concept of medicine as a profession introduced into the history of medical ethics in the eighteenth century by these two remarkable physician-ethicists has proven to be both durable and clinically applicable today. The professional responsibility model of perinatal ethics protects clinical judgment and practice from the simplistic, clinically inadequate alternatives of maternal rights-based reductionism and fetal rights-based reductionism. The professional responsibility model does so by requiring, in all cases, deliberative consideration of beneficence-based and autonomy-based obligations to the pregnant patient and beneficence-based obligations to the fetal patient. The informed consent process should be used as a preventive ethics tool to empower pregnant women to make informed, deliberative, and voluntary decisions.

In the chapters that follow, we will deploy the professional responsibility model of perinatal ethics to address comprehensively the ethical challenges that perinatologists confront in clinical practice and research. These chapters will demonstrate the practicality of the professional responsibility model of perinatal ethics.

1.5 References

1. Chervenak FA, McCullough LB. Clinical guides to preventing ethical conflicts between pregnant women and their physicians. Am J Obstet Gynecol 1990;162:303–307.
2. McCullough LB, Chervenak FA. Ethics in Obstetrics and Gynecology. New York, NY: Oxford University Press, 1994.
3. Chervenak FA, McCullough LB, Brent RL. The professional responsibility model of obstetric ethics: avoiding the perils of clashing rights. Am J Obstet Gynecol 2011;205:315.e1–5.
4. Engelhardt HT Jr. The Foundations of Bioethics. 2nd ed. New York, NY: Oxford University Press, 1995.
5. Beauchamp TL, Childress JF. Principles of Biomedical Ethics. 6th ed. New York, NY: Oxford University Press, 2009.
6. Hippocrates. Oath of Hippocrates. In: Temkin O, Temkin CL, eds. Ancient Medicine: Selected Papers of Ludwig Edelstein, p. 6. Baltimore, MD: Johns Hopkins University Press 1976:6.
7. Faden RR, Beauchamp TL. A History and Theory of Informed Consent. New York, NY: Oxford University Press, 1986.
8. McCullough LB, Coverdale JH, Chervenak FA. Ethical challenges of decision making with pregnant patients who have schizophrenia. Am J Obstet Gynecol 2002;187:696–702.
9. Schloendorff v. The Society of The New York Hospital, 211 N.Y. 125, 126, 105 N.E. 92, 93 (1914).
10. Brett AS, McCullough LB. When patients request specific interventions: Defining the limits of the physician's obligation. N Engl J Med 1986;315:1347–51.

11. Brett AS, McCullough LB. Addressing requests by patients for non-beneficial interventions. JAMA 2012:307:149–50.
12. Callahan S, Callahan D, eds. Abortion: Understanding Differences. New York, NY: Plenum Press, 1984.
13. Strong C. Ethics in Reproductive and Perinatal Medicine. New Haven, CT: Yale University Press, 1997.
14. Annas GJ. Protecting the liberty of pregnant patient. N Engl J Med 1988;316:1213–1214.
15. Ruddick W, Wilcox W. Operating on the fetus. Hastings Cent Report 1982;12:10–14.
16. Chervenak FA, McCullough LB. The limits of viability. J Perinat Med 1997;25:418–20.
17. Chervenak FA, McCullough LB, Levene MI. An ethically justified clinically comprehensive approach to periviability: gynaecological, obstetric, perinatal, and neonatal dimensions. J Obstet Gynaecol 2007;27:3–7.
18. American Academy of Pediatrics, Committee on Bioethics. Informed consent, parental permission, and assent in pediatric practice. Pediatrics 1995;95:314–317.
19. Saigal S, Tyson J. Measurement of quality of life of survivors of neonatal intensive care: critique and implications. Semin Perinatol 2008;32:59–66.
20. Johnson LSM. Abortion: II. Contemporary ethical and legal aspects: A. ethical perspectives. In Post SG (ed) Encyclopedia of Bioethics, pp. 7–18. New York: Macmillan References USA, 2004.
21. Lyerly AD, Little MO. Toward an ethically responsible approach to vaginal birth after cesarean. Semin Perinatol 2010;34:337–344.
22. Minkoff H, Paltrow L. Obstetricians and the rights of pregnant women. Womens Health (Lond Engl) 2007;3:315–319.
23. Högberg U, Lynöe N, Wulff M. Cesarean by choice? Empirical study of public attitudes. Acta Obstet Gynecol Scand 2008;87:1301–1308.
24. Buckley S. Reclaiming every woman's birthright. Midwifery Today Int Midwife 2010;94:40–41.
25. Minkoff H. NIH Vaginal Birth after Cesarean: New Insights. National Institutes of Health Consensus Development Conference, March 10–13, 2010. Page 6, Day 2 Discussion, available at http://videocast.nih.gov/summary.asp?Live=8408, accessed June 19, 2014.
26. McCullough LB. The ethical concept of medicine as a profession: its origins in modern medical ethics and implications for physicians. In Kenny N, Shelton W (eds) Lost Virtue: Professional Character Development in Medical Education, pp. 17–27. New York: Elsevier, 2006.
27. Chervenak FA, McCullough LB, Grünebaum A, Arabin B, Levene MI, Brent RL. Planned home birth in the United States and professionalism: a critical assessment. J Clin Ethics. 2013 Fall;24(3):184–91.

1.6 Summary points

- To implement the professional responsibility model of perinatal ethics in clinical practice and research, the perinatologist must, in all cases, identify and balance beneficence-based and autonomy-based obligations to the pregnant woman and beneficence-based obligations to the fetal patient.
- The perinatologist should engage the pregnant woman in the informed consent process to empower her to make informed, deliberative, and voluntary decisions about the clinical management of pregnancy and participation in clinical research.
- The perinatologist should engage the parents of the neonatal patient in the informed consent process, to empower them to make informed, deliberative,

and voluntary decisions about the clinical management of child and participation in clinical research.

- Directive counseling for the clinical benefit of the fetal or pregnant patient, when supported in deliberative clinical ethical judgment, is ethically justified in the informed consent process about the management of pregnancy.
- Delivery makes an ethical difference: Perinatal ethics during pregnancy and after delivery differ because the ethical concepts of being a fetal patient and being a neonatal patient differ significantly.
- Directive counseling for clinical benefit of the neonatal patient in the informed consent process with parents should be guided by the best interests of the child standard.
- Rights-based reductionism is an inadequate basis for perinatal ethics in clinical practice and research, and therefore should be abandoned.

2 Induced abortion and feticide

2.1 Introduction

Induced abortion and feticide continue to be ethically controversial and challenging in obstetric practice.[1,2] While the American Medical Association[3–8] and the American College of Obstetricians and Gynecologists[9–12] provide general ethical guidance, the professional responsibility model of perinatal ethics provides practical, comprehensive, ethical guidance for physicians on when to offer, recommend, perform, and refer pregnant patients for induced abortion or feticide.[13]

2.2 Terminology

"Abortion" and "feticide" are often used without precision. Failure to be clear about their precise meanings hobbles any attempt at ethical analysis.

"Abortion" and "feticide" have precise, descriptive, medical meanings. When used with precision, they can and should be distinguished from each other. According to Stedman's Medical Dictionary, abortion is the "[e]xpulsion from the uterus of an embryo or fetus before viability."[14] Abortion can occur spontaneously or be induced. Induced abortion, because it occurs before viability, will result in the death of the embryo(s) or fetus(es). Feticide is defined as the "[d]estruction of the embryo or fetus in the uterus"[14] independently of gestational age and is not determinative whether the uterus is emptied. Feticide can be performed by such means as injection of potassium chloride or ligation of the umbilical cord.[10,15] "Multifetal pregnancy reduction" is the use of feticide to cause the death of embryo(s) or fetus(es), which typically remains in the ongoing pregnancy.[10] The more precise terminology is "selective feticide," because of the vagueness of the word "reduction," especially for lay audiences. Termination of pregnancy is the "[i]nduced ending of a pregnancy"[14] independently of gestational age and is not determinative whether survival occurs. In light of this definition, "selective termination" can be confusing and should not be used, because selective feticide does not end the pregnancy of the surviving fetus(es).

In this chapter, we use "induced abortion" rather than simply "abortion" to be precise that spontaneous abortion is not included. We use "feticide" with the descriptive meaning above. Both "induced abortion" and "feticide" are value-neutral, medical terms.

2.3 Offering induced during abortion or feticide

2.3.1 After viability

The concept of a serious fetal anomaly is essential to the application of the professional responsibility model to induced abortion and feticide after viability. "Serious fetal anomaly" means that there is a certain or near certain diagnosis of an anomaly that is reliably expected either to result in death, even with aggressive obstetric and neonatal intervention, or short-term survival with severe and irreversible deficit of cognitive developmental capacity. In Chapter 3, we show that induced abortion of fetuses of 24 weeks gestational age and later without serious fetal anomalies is not ethically permissible. After viability, i.e. throughout the third trimester of pregnancy, there is a beneficence-based prohibition against feticide of viable fetuses without serious anomalies, because the beneficence-based obligation to protect the life and health of the fetal patient remains intact; its limits have not been reached. As a consequence, both the physician and the pregnant woman have beneficence-based obligations to protect the health and life of the viable fetal patient without severe anomalies. It follows that it is ethically impermissible to offer feticide for viable fetuses without anomalies or with less-than-severe anomalies, such as Down syndrome or achondroplasia. Less-than-severe anomalies do not involve a high probability of death or a high probability of the absence or virtual absence of cognitive developmental capacity.[15,16]

When a viable fetus has a severe anomaly, offering feticide followed by termination of pregnancy is ethically appropriate. This is because the beneficence-based obligation to protect the life of the fetus that has been diagnosed with a severe anomaly has reached its limits: the outcomes of death or of short-term survival with severe and irreversible deficit of cognitive developmental capacity cannot be prevented.[15,16]

2.3.2 Before viability

There are two beneficence-based justifications for offering induced abortion before viability. The first is based on a deliberative clinical judgment that continued pregnancy poses a threat to the health or life of the pregnant woman. Pre-existing conditions, such as severe cardiac disease or some forms of cancer, can pose such threats.[17] When the best available evidence supports the clinical judgment that continued pregnancy poses a risk to the pregnant woman's health or life, she should be informed about this matter and offered the alternative of induced abortion. It is important to appreciate that this beneficence-based justification will evolve over time as new evidence accumulates about the risks of pregnancy to women from pre-existing conditions or the complications of pregnancy. Some women, because of moral convictions about the general moral status of the fetus, will refuse this offer. They should be informed that their refusal increases the risk that their health could be severely compromised and that they could die. The final decision to remain pregnant or to elect induced abortion is ultimately a function of the pregnant woman's autonomy and should be respected by the physician.

The second beneficence-based justification for offering feticide before viability is based on reliable clinical judgment that continued pregnancy poses a threat to the life or health of co-existent fetuses, such as is the case in higher-order pregnancies and twin pregnancies in which the continued existence of the anomalous fetus that is causing hydramnios poses a threat to the health or life of the other fetus. Current evidence supports the clinical judgment that these risks can be reduced by selective feticide.[10] When the best available evidence supports the clinical judgment that continued multifetal, previable pregnancy poses a risk to the other fetus' or fetuses' health or life, the pregnant woman should be informed about this matter and offered the alternative of selective feticide. Some women, because of moral convictions about the general moral status of the fetus, will refuse this offer. They should be informed that their refusal increases the risk that the pregnancy will end before viability without any surviving fetuses or end prematurely after viability, with increased risk of infant mortality and morbidity. The final decision to remain pregnant, to elect induced abortion, or to elect selective feticide is ultimately a function of the pregnant woman's autonomy and should be respected by the physician.

When the best available evidence supports the deliberative clinical judgment that continued previable pregnancy does not pose an increased risk to the health or life of the pregnant woman or fetuses, the only remaining justification for offering induced abortion or feticide is autonomy-based. There are five clinical circumstances in which induced abortion should be offered. First, some pregnant women will request an induced abortion. Second, a previable pregnancy will be diagnosed with an anomaly or viable pregnancy will be diagnosed with a severe anomaly. Third, a complication occurs that threatens the successful continuation of a previable pregnancy, such as preterm premature rupture of membranes. Fourth, a complication may be present in pregnancy that jeopardizes maternal health or life, such as cancer or severe eclampsia. Fifth, some pregnant women will directly, and sometimes indirectly, express concern about remaining pregnant or will be concerned about multiple birth and will prefer for economic or other personal reasons to have a singleton pregnancy. Physicians should respond to these five groups by discussing the option of induced abortion and, when appropriate, explaining time limitations.

In response to the offer of induced abortion, physicians should expect pregnant women to sort themselves into three sub-groups.[18] Some will want to continue the pregnancy because they decide to accept whatever child results. Some will not want to remain pregnant and will elect induced abortion. Some will be uncertain about whether to continue the pregnancy. Respecting the autonomy of pregnant women means that physicians should respect this self-sorting, by limiting their role to providing information in a non-directive fashion (offering but not recommending induced abortion) that these women can use to resolve their uncertainty. Attempting to bias woman's decision assumes, falsely, that physicians have the professional competence to decide for a woman with a previable pregnancy that she should or should not remain pregnant.

Non-directive counseling should guide physicians in discussing induced abortion with women with previable pregnancies who remain uncertain. Physicians should refrain from making, suggesting, or implying a recommendation about continuation or termination of a previable pregnancy. Directive counseling toward continuation of a previable pregnancy based on alleged benefit to the pregnant woman of providing information about fetal development or showing images of fetal development, to prevent remorse or regret, lacks an evidence base. Such directive counseling is an ethically impermissible distortion of the physician's professional role in the informed consent process.[19] All women should be informed that their decision about termination is time-limited, given the availability of induced abortion. In addition, in order to respect autonomy, the physician should provide frank, evidence-based information about maternal or fetal conditions, even if it is emotionally distressing. Physicians need to make the time available for the sometimes extensive and iterative discussions required to disclose the medical facts and assist the woman to assimilate those medical facts into her decision-making process.

Pregnant women who elect induced abortion or feticide should be assured that ethical and legal obligations of confidentiality will be fulfilled: Others will be informed about the patient's decision only with her explicit permission or, in the case of minors, as required by applicable law.[4] In particular, should she elect absolute confidentiality, her husband or partner should not be informed. Again, physicians have no professional competence in this matter, and therefore should respect the pregnant woman's autonomous decisions about whom she wants informed by the physician.

Individual conscience, i.e. the values and beliefs of a physician that arise from sources outside the ethical concept of medicine as a profession, such as upbringing and religion, does not justifiably place limits on the ethics of offering induced abortion or feticide when the above ethical justifications apply. There are two reasons why this is the case. The first is that every physician's obligation to provide appropriate information in the informed consent process is a matter of professional responsibility, not individual conscience. Second, one cannot predict how women will sort themselves in response to offering induced abortion or feticide. Subsequent decisions are a function ultimately of the pregnant woman's autonomy. It is, therefore, a mistake to think that offering induced abortion or feticide makes the physician somehow responsible for the informed, deliberative, and voluntary decisions of a pregnant patient that may not be consistent with the physician's individual conscience, because the physician's offer does not control the pregnant woman's decision-making process; she controls it.[20]

2.4 Recommending induced abortion or feticide

There are four categories for which recommendations of induced abortion or feticide are considered. The first is when a maternal condition, or treatment of such a condition, results in increased risk to the pregnant woman's health or life should she continue her pregnancy. The second is when continued pregnancy without induced abortion or feticide substantially increases the risk to the health or life of fetus(es). The third is for feticide when a serious anomaly has been diagnosed. The fourth occurs in complications that threaten the woman's health or life and salvage of the fetus is clinically hopeless. We will argue that recommendations are not ethically justified for the first three, but only for the fourth.

The first and second categories can be addressed together. The first requires balancing the life and health of the pregnant woman against the health and life of the fetal patient in rare cases, such as some forms of cancer[17] or mirror syndrome. The second category requires balancing the life and health of multiple fetal patients. These judgments, at first, appear to be purely beneficence-based, and therefore within the scope of the physician's professional competence to make recommendations, but on closer examination are not. This is because these judgments involve deciding which health or life is more important. This is ultimately not a beneficence-based judgment but autonomy-based, appealing to the cultural, religious, and other individual beliefs of the pregnant woman. Respecting the pregnant woman's autonomy means that the physician should be non-directive and not seek to bias the woman's decision-making process, e.g. by "soft pedaling" the benefits or overemphasizing the risks of continued pregnancy. No recommendation of induced abortion or feticide is ethically justified when the woman is undecided about how to balance her and the fetal patient's interests. Individual conscience is not implicated because physicians are not responsible for the ultimate balancing judgments that pregnant women will make in these tragic circumstances after they been informed about them by their physician.[17]

Third, given the nature of severe fetal anomalies, one might think that recommendation of induced abortion or feticide would be justified, e.g. for anencephaly or trisomy 13. Women with serious moral convictions about the moral status of the fetus, especially women with religious convictions about the sanctity of fetal life, will experience a recommendation of induced abortion or feticide as profoundly disrespectful of their autonomy. They may experience moral distress when offered this alternative but offering an alternative, while distressful, is not profoundly disrespectful of the conscience and convictions of such pregnant women and is, therefore, ethically permissible.

The fourth category is straightforward in beneficence-based clinical judgment. For complications such as preterm premature rupture of membranes with chorioamnionitis, the fetal condition is hopeless clinically and the woman's health, and perhaps life, is in danger. There is, therefore, no beneficence-based obligation to the fetus, and there is a strong beneficence-based obligation to the pregnant woman to protect her health or life, which justifies a recommendation for induced abortion.

2.5 Performing induced abortion or feticide

There are two major ethical issues concerning performing induced abortion or feticide. The first concerns the method of terminating the pregnancy. The second concerns whether individual conscience places ethically justified barriers on an individual physician's performing induced abortion or feticide.

Before viability, it is ethically permissible in professional medical ethics, and therefore in professional conscience, to perform an induced abortion. This is because, as explained above, the pregnant woman is free to withhold or withdraw the moral status of being a patient from the previable fetus at her discretion. Induced abortion of the previable fetus in such circumstances, therefore, does not involve the killing of a patient and is permissible in professional medical ethics.[19] For the same reason, performing feticide in a previable pregnancy is ethically permissible in professional medical ethics.

Pregnant women should not be presumed to understand that expelling the near-viable fetus or a viable fetus with a severe anomaly from the uterus could result in a live birth and that feticide can prevent this outcome. In such circumstances, live birth creates an increased risk of preventable neonatal morbidity. There is a beneficence-based obligation of the physician and the pregnant woman to prevent this risk. Refusal of feticide can also be seen as contradictory because election of termination of pregnancy means that the pregnant woman does not wish to have a child issue from her current pregnancy. Such contradictory thinking is evidence of significant impairment of autonomous decision making. In such a setting, it is reasonable for the physician to require that the pregnant woman accept feticide as a condition for performing termination of her pregnancy. Performing feticide in this setting also exonerates the physician from being accused of performing a so-called "partial-birth abortion." The correct account is that the physician is evacuating the uterus after ethically justified iatrogenic fetal demise.

In the United States, "partial-birth abortion" has been prohibited by state law, a prohibition upheld by the U. S. Supreme Court.[21] We emphasize that "partial-birth abortion" is a purely political phrase and should never become part of medical discourse.[22] "Partial-birth abortion" describes feticide that is employed in the course of emptying the uterus rather than before the uterus is emptied. There is no special ethical challenge involved, because the above analysis of feticide before and after viability applies. Laws prohibiting "partial-birth abortion" represent an ethically unjustified intrusion into professional medical practice.[23]

Some physicians may have objections in individual conscience to participation in induced abortion or feticide. Respecting individual conscience means that such physicians should be free to refuse to perform induced abortion or feticide. An important implication of this analysis of individual conscience is that a requirement of residents or fellows to participate in induced abortion or feticide is ethically impermissible. However, a requirement that trainees have an appropriate fund of knowledge about these procedures and an appropriate fund of knowledge and clinical skills in managing their complications is consistent with individual conscience and a matter of professional obligation.[19]

Physicians with individual-conscience-based objections to induced abortion or feticide must keep in mind, when they refuse to perform the procedure, that individual conscience does *not* govern the physician's professional role. It is, therefore, impermissible for the physician, on the basis of individual conscience, to express judgments about the morality of a woman's election of induced abortion or feticide, or of colleagues who perform these procedures, because doing so is inconsistent with non-directive counseling regarding induced abortion before viability.[19]

The obligation of a community to ensure access to termination of pregnancy involves complex and controversial appeals to social justice that are beyond the scope of this chapter. While it could be argued that every community has such a social-justice based obligation, social justice itself requires respect for individual conscience and cannot, therefore, mandate violations of individual conscience. An important exception is termination for pregnancy for maternal indications in a medical emergency, such as obstetric hemorrhage or severe intrauterine infection, conditions for which there is no time to transfer the care of the pregnant woman to another physician or facility.

2.6 Referring for induced abortion or feticide

The ethics of referral for induced abortion or feticide is straightforward for physicians who do not have conscience-based objections to induced abortion. They can make what we call direct referrals.[23] The referring physician sees to it that the patient will be seen by a colleague competent and willing to perform the procedure.

Direct referral appears not to be an option for physicians with a conscience-based objection to induced abortion or feticide, because of the explicit involvement of the physician in the subsequent termination of a pregnancy. To concomitantly respect the pregnant woman's autonomy and the individual conscience of physicians opposed to induced abortion or feticide, an indirect referral for termination of pregnancy should be made. Indirect referral is both autonomy-based and beneficence-based. When it is obligatory to offer induced abortion or feticide, respect for the pregnant woman's autonomy in previable pregnancies requires the physician to inform her that induced abortion or feticide is an option. Beneficence requires the physician to provide information about clinics or agencies, such as Planned Parenthood in the United States, that provide competent and safe induced abortion or feticide. The physician's individual conscience is not violated, because whether an induced abortion or feticide subsequently occurs is solely a function of the pregnant woman's autonomy after she visits the clinic or agency of her own accord. The referring physician is, therefore, not responsible for a subsequent induced abortion or feticide. In summary, direct referral for induced abortion or feticide is not ethically required but is ethically permissible. Conscience-based objections to direct referral for induced abortion or feticide have merit; conscience-based objections to indirect referral do not.[23]

2.7 Conclusion

The professional responsibility model of perinatal ethics provides guidance for decision making about offering, recommending, performing, and referring for induced abortion or feticide. The result is a comprehensive account that respects autonomy-based and beneficence-based obligations to the pregnant woman, beneficence-based obligations to the fetal patient, the professional responsibility of physicians, and the individual conscience of physicians opposed to induced abortion or feticide. The physician's role in offering, recommending, performing, and referring for induced abortion or feticide is based primarily on professional responsibility, shaped by autonomy-based and beneficence-based obligations of the physician, with important but limited constraints originating in individual conscience.

2.8 References

1. Johnson LSM. Abortion II: contemporary ethical and legal aspects: A. ethical perspectives. In Post SG, ed. Encyclopedia of Bioethics, 3rd ed. New York: Macmillan Reference USA, 2004:7–18.
2. Allen AL. Abortion II: contemporary ethical and legal aspects: B. legal and regulatory issues. In Post SG, ed. Encyclopedia of Bioethics, 3rd ed. New York: Macmillan Reference USA, 2004:18–28.
3. American Medical Association. E-201 Abortion. Available at www0.ama-assn.org/apps/pf_new/pf_online?f_n=browse&doc=policyfiles/HnE/E-2.01.HTM&&s_t=&st_p=&nth=1&prev_pol=policyfiles/HnE/E-1.02.HTM&nxt_pol=policyfiles/HnE/E-2.01.HTM&. Accessed March 8, 2014.
4. American Medical Association. E-5.05 Confidentiality. Available at www0.ama-assn.org/apps/pf_new/pf_online?f_n=browse&doc=policyfiles/HnE/E-5.05.HTM&&s_t=&st_p=&nth=1&prev_pol=policyfiles/HnE/E-4.07.HTM&nxt_pol=policyfiles/HnE/E-5.01.HTM&. Accessed March 8, 2014.
5. American Medical Association. H-5.983. Pregnancy Termination. Available at www0.ama-assn.org/apps/pf_new/pf_online?f_n=browse&n_p=T&&s_t=&st_p=&nth=1&prev_pol=policyfiles/HnE/H-5.988.HTM&nxt_pol=policyfiles/HnE/H-5.990.HTM&. Accessed March 8, 2014.
6. American Medical Association. H-5.990 Policy on Abortion. Available at www0.ama-assn.org/apps/pf_new/pf_online?f_n=browse&p_p=T&&s_t=&st_p=&nth=1&prev_pol=policyfiles/HnE/H-5.990.HTM&nxt_pol=policyfiles/HnE/H-5.992.HTM&. Accessed March 8, 2014.
7. American Medical Association. H-5.993 Right to Privacy in Termination of Pregnancy. Available at www.ama-assn.org/apps/pf_new/pf_online?f_n=browse&doc=policyfiles/HnE/H-5.993.HTM&&s_t=&st_p=&nth=1&prev_pol=policyfiles/HOD-TOC.HTM&nxt_pol=policyfiles/HnE/H-5.982.HTM&. Accessed March 8, 2014.
8. American Medical Association. H-5995. Abortion. Available at www.ama-assn.org/apps/pf_new/pf_online?f_n=browse&doc=policyfiles/HnE/H-5.995.HTM&&s_t=&st_p=&nth=1&prev_

pol=policyfiles/HOD-TOC.HTM&nxt_pol=policyfiles/HnE/H-5.982.HTM&. Accessed March 8, 2014.

9. American College of Obstetricians and Gynecologists. Committee on Practice Bulletins. Medical management of abortion. Clinical management guidelines for obstetrician-gynecologists number 67. Obstet Gynecol 2005;106:871–882.
10. American College of Obstetricians and Gynecologists. Committee on Ethics. Multifetal Pregnancy Reduction. ACOG committee opinion number 369. Obstet Gynecol 2007;109:1511–1515.
11. American College of Obstetricians and Gynecologists Statement of Policy. Executive Board. Abortion policy. Reaffirmed July 2011. Available at http://www.physiciansforreproductiverights.org/wp-content/uploads/2013/03/ACOG-abortion-policy.pdf, accessed June 19, 2014.
12. American College of Obstetricians and Gynecologists. Committee on Ethics. The limits of conscientious refusal in reproductive medicine. Opinion Number 385. Obstet Gynecol 2007;110:1203–1208.
13. Chervenak FA, McCullough LB. An ethically justified, practical approach to offering, recommending, performing, and referring for induced abortion and infanticide. Am J Obstet Gynecol 2009;201:560.e1–6.
14. Stedman's Medical Dictionary. Available at online.statref.com/DictionaryHelp/DictionaryHelp.aspx?type=dictionary&SessionId=E64234MHHTKYZGGZ&prnt=dlo&chwin=false, accessed March 8, 2014.
15. Chervenak FA, McCullough LB, Campbell S. Is third trimester abortion justified? Brit J Obstet Gynaecol. 1995;102:434–435.
16. Chervenak FA, McCullough LB, Campbell S. Third trimester abortion: Is compassion enough? Brit J Obstet Gynæcol 1999;106:293–296.
17. Chervenak FA, McCullough LB, Knapp RC, Caputo TA, Barber HR. A clinically comprehensive ethical framework for offering and recommending cancer treatment before and during pregnancy. Cancer 2004 Jan 15;100(2):215–222.
18. Chervenak FA, McCullough LB, Sharma G, Davis J, Gross S. Enhancing patient autonomy with risk assessment and invasive diagnosis: an ethical solution to a clinical challenge. Am J Obstet Gynecol 2008;199:19.e1–4.
19. McCullough LB, Chervenak FA. Ethics in Obstetrics and Gynecology. New York: Oxford University Press, 1994.
20. Thorp JM, Wells SR, Bowes WA Jr., Cefalo RC. Integrity, abortion, and the pro-life perinatologist. Hastings Cent Rep 1995;25:27–28.
21. Annas GJ. "Partial-birth abortion" and the Supreme Court. N Engl J Med 2001;344:152–156.
22. American Medical Association. Council on Ethical and Judicial Affairs. H-5.982 Late-Term Pregnancy Termination Techniques. Available at www.ama-assn.org/apps/pf_new/pf_online?f_n=browse&doc=policyfiles/HnE/H-5.982.HTM. Accessed March 8, 2014.
23. Chervenak FA, McCullough LB. The ethics of direct and indirect referral for termination of pregnancy. Am J Obstet Gynecol 2008;199:232.e1–232.e3.

2.9 Summary points

- When a viable fetus has a severe anomaly, offering feticide, followed by termination of pregnancy, is ethically appropriate.
- Before viability, it is appropriate to offer induced abortion when continuing the pregnancy threatens the health or life of the pregnant woman or the life or health of co-existent fetuses.

- Before viability, it is appropriate to offer induced abortion when the pregnant woman requests it, she expresses concern about remaining pregnant, the fetus is diagnosed with an anomaly, a complication threatens the successful completion of the pregnancy, or when a complication jeopardizes the life or health of the pregnant woman.
- It is ethically permissible to perform induced abortion or feticide before viability.
- It is ethically permissible to perform feticide before induced abortion for a serious fetal anomaly diagnosed periviably or after viabilility.
- Physicians, who have an individual-conscience-based objection to induced abortion or feticide, are not ethically obligated to perform either procedure but are ethically obligated to make an indirect referral.

3 Periviability

3.1 Introduction

Periviability, 22–26 completed weeks gestational age, has generated ongoing clinical ethical controversies concerning the roles of abortion, cesarean delivery for fetal indication, neonatal resuscitation, and limits on life-sustaining treatment of neonates.[1–4] This chapter provides an ethically justified, clinically comprehensive approach to the management of periviability in its obstetric and neonatal dimensions.[5,6] Deliberative clinical ethical judgment should be guided by outcomes data when they are available.

3.2 Clinical outcomes data

It is important to consider regional outcomes data of infants born in the post-surfactant era (after the early 1990s), including infants born alive who died before admission to the NICU. Levene has presented consolidated data on studies fulfilling these criteria and has interpolated rates of major disability by gestational age interval from 22–26 weeks. Major disability was defined as cerebral palsy affecting independent locomotion, IQ <70, or severe visual impairment and deafness requiring hearing aids.[7]

When these data are compared with similar published studies but based on a single center of excellence and applying the same criteria as the geographically based studies, there is a difference in adverse outcome for the most immature babies. Babies born in "centers of excellence" have a better outcome than babies of similar gestational ages from geographically based studies. The extent of this difference for the most immature infants of <25 weeks gestation is equivalent to the advantage of being born one week earlier in a "center of excellence" compared with a unit within a geographically base cohort. Therefore, an intact outcome for a baby born at 24 weeks of gestation in a center of excellence is equivalent to the rate of intact survival for a baby born in a geographically based cohort at 25 weeks. Survival without any such major disability at 22 and 23 weeks is very low in all studies, whether center of excellence or geographically based. Data from geographically based data show that less than 25 % of babies born alive at 24 weeks survive without major disability,[7] but the same risk of bad outcome reported from centers of excellence is 23 weeks.

Two studies have reported outcomes within a recent 10 year period to establish whether there has been improvement in the post-surfactant era of perinatal care. Data from the American NICHD network showed that outcomes among infants of <25 weeks gestational age are not improving despite more aggressive perinatal and neonatal treatment.[8] A similar study of all babies born <25 weeks in the state of Victoria, Australia found that 15 % survived without major disability in the presurfactant era compared with 23 % in the post-surfactant era. Further analysis of this study shows that for every 10 surviving infants in the first era, only 5 were severely disabled compared to 8 for every 10 "healthy" survivors in the later era, indicating improved outcomes.[9]

3.3 Induced abortion

Advances in perinatal medicine have resulted in mortality and morbidity being reduced in tandem for fetuses at or above 24 weeks with the proportion of intact survivors being equal to or greater than the proportion of survivors with significant functional impairments. This simultaneous reduction of mortality and morbidity supports the beneficence-based clinical judgment that the outcomes of perinatal intervention for this population of periviable fetuses results in a greater balance of clinical goods over clinical harms. These outcomes data also support the justice-based clinical judgment that the proportion of intact to injured survivors is fair; there is no maldistribution of the benefits and harms of clinical intervention in this population that result in exploitation. Induced abortion is, therefore, not an ethically acceptable option at 24 weeks and above in the absence of lethal or other very serious anomalies.[10] (See also Chapter 2)

At 22 weeks or before, mortality reaches 100 %, which means that perinatal intervention for this patient population would be futile in terms of survival. Neither beneficence-based nor justice-based obligations of the physician are violated by abortion of such periviable fetuses. Induced abortion is therefore an ethically acceptable option at 22 weeks or before.

At 23 weeks the percent of survivors is significantly below 50 %, while even fewer survive without severe disability, compared to disability rates at 24 weeks or later. There is a marked disproportion of survivors with major disability to intact survivors.[7,11] This means, in justice-based clinical judgment, that the outcomes are unfair because exploitation occurs: only a very small percent of infants experience the benefit of survival with intact functional status while the vast majority either dies or survives with significant impairments. While the Victoria study indicates improved outcomes in the more recent cohort, there is nonetheless a mortality rate of 59 % and 6 % survivors with severe disability, for a total of 65 %[9] burdened with no opportunity for offsetting clinical benefit because death and severe disability are irreversible. The latter two groups experience only the burdens of intervention with no opportunity to experience offsetting clinical benefit, which is incompatible with the requirements of justice applied to clinical outcomes data.[1]

An observational report from the Vermont-Oxford network stated that for the 23-week population neonatal intervention involves an "uncontrolled experiment."[12] This judgment has the important ethical implication that aggressive management should not be regarded as the standard of care. The pregnant woman is therefore ethically free to withdraw the moral status of being a patient from such a fetus and requesting abortion. Induced abortion is therefore an ethically acceptable option at 23 weeks. In our view, feticide is advisable in such cases, because the fetus is no longer a patient.

For some fetuses, the presence of serious anomalies may result in very poor outcomes, which resemble those of fetuses at an earlier gestational age, depending on the severity of the anomaly.[7] “Serious fetal anomaly” means that there is a certain or near certain diagnosis of an anomaly that is reliably expected either to result in death, even with aggressive obstetric and neonatal intervention, or short-term survival with severe and irreversible deficit of cognitive developmental capacity. Beneficence-based clinical judgment should be based on the best available evidence about outcomes for these anomalies. Abortion of such fetuses is ethically permissible. (See Chapter 2)

For other fetuses in the 23–24 week range, it is essential to do the best gestational age assessment and then apply the most pertinent gestational-age based ethical analysis. When in vitro fertilization has occurred, gestational age can be reliably determined to within plus or minus one day. With high quality ultrasound evaluation, gestational age can be reliably determined to within plus or minus one week.[13]

3.4 Obstetric and neonatal dimensions

The clinical management of pregnancies involving a periviable fetus, the goal of which is live birth, has obstetric and neonatal components. Such management should be understood as a lead-in to critical-care management of the fetal and neonatal patient, with cesarean delivery the first step toward critical care intervention. This first step is followed, in the case of live birth, by resuscitation and admission to the neonatal intensive care unit for the administration of ongoing life-sustaining treatment.

Critical-care management of life-threatening conditions should in all cases be understood as a trial of intervention that has two goals. The first goal is short-term, to prevent imminent death. The second goal is long-term, survival with minimized morbidity and maximized functional status. A trial means just that: clinical intervention should be initiated and continued only so long as it is reasonable to expect that its goals will be accomplished in deliberative clinical ethical judgment. When either goal of critical care can no longer reasonably be expected to be accomplished, the ethical obligation to continue the trial ends.

For fetuses at 22 weeks and earlier, imminent death cannot be prevented and the woman is, therefore, subjected to surgical management with no offsetting clinical benefit for the fetal patient. For this population, neither cesarean delivery nor resuscitation should be offered for neonatal benefit and, if requested, should be refused on the basis of futility in terms of survival of the fetal patient.

For fetuses at 24 weeks gestational age or later, without severe fetal anomalies, perinatal interventions should be initiated when the best available evidence indicates that they will improve outcomes. Cesarean delivery for fetal indications, such as fetal distress, and immediate neonatal resuscitation in this population are two such perinatal interventions. This is because they are necessary to achieve the short-term goal of critical care, preventing the imminent death of the neonate, and have a reasonable probability of achieving the long-term goal.

For fetuses at 23 weeks, we again refer to the conclusion of the Vermont-Oxford network report that neonatal intervention involves an uncontrolled experiment.[12] In the language of beneficence, this means that the outcomes do not clearly involve a greater balance of clinical goods over harms and may, indeed, involve the opposite. In the latter case, justice would be violated.

These outcomes do support the conclusion that the short-term goal of perinatal intervention can be accomplished. Such intervention is not futile in terms of preventing imminent death. However, these outcomes also support the clinical ethical judgment that life-sustaining neonatal treatment may later become futile in terms of long-term survival. These outcomes, especially if they involve a disproportion of burdens to benefits, also support the clinical ethical judgment that life-sustaining neonatal treatment may later also become futile in terms of acceptable functional status. These clinical ethical judgments mean that the burden of proof, which usually falls on those who wish to limit treatment, may fall equally on those who wish to provide and those who wish to limit treatment or, indeed, only on those who wish to provide treatment. It follows that the physician should only offer but not recommend perinatal intervention, including resuscitation. Well informed parental requests for such intervention should be implemented, emphasizing the concept of a trial of intervention. The patient populations for which such intervention may be worth considering can be defined more precisely by using the decision-making tool demonstrated by Tyson et al. to be reliable for neonatal patients[14] but which Skupski et al. have shown not to be reliable in obstetric clinical judgment.[15]

Beneficence-based and justice-based considerations are relevant to setting ethically justified limits on neonatal intervention. It is well accepted that neonatal critical care may be discontinued when the patient has a terminal or irreversible condition, as defined in applicable advance directive legislation.

It is also recognized that prolonged resuscitation can become futile in terms of its intended physiologic outcome, the restoration of spontaneous circulation. There are accepted criteria for invoking physiologic futility to discontinue neonatal resuscitation.[16,17] Neonatal life-sustaining treatment can become futile in one or more of several senses.[18] (See Chapter 9) Physiologic futility exists when there is no reasonable expectation that the physiological outcome of clinical management will occur, e.g. when maximum mechanical ventilatory support for a neonatal patients results in levels of oxygenation not compatible with life. The concept of imminent demise futility means that the patient is not expected to survive to discharge and has such serious neurologic injury or loss that the patient will never gain or regain the capacity to interact with the environment and grow and develop as a human being. The concept of clinical or overall futility means that, while the patient is expected to survive, the patient has irreversibly lost the capacity to interact with the environment and grow and develop as a human being.

In some cases, none of these concepts of futility apply. At the same time, there is growing concern that continuing neonatal life-sustaining treatment is increasingly unlikely to achieve the second goal of critical care. We characterize such cases as those for which there is not yet a sufficient clinical basis for a beneficence-based clinical judgment to discontinue such treatment while, at the same time, the beneficence-based obligation to continue is not robust. The ethical concern here is that disease-related and iatrogenic burdens on the patient continue to mount while the downward course appears ever more irreversible. The Jesuit moral theologian, Richard McCormick, one of the founders of the field of bioethics, argued that we should understand such cases in the following terms. Sometimes, the expected progression of disease and the increasingly limited effects of treatment combine to result in disease-related and iatrogenic burdens that overwhelm the small remaining developmental capacity. It is not at all clear that there is a beneficence-based obligation to a patient to continue neonatal life-sustaining treatment.[19] When we consider the population of patients whose remaining developmental capacity has been overwhelmed, continued treatment may begin to violate justice. In such cases, offering parents the alternative of discontinuing life-sustaining treatment becomes, in our view, ethically acceptable.

Parents who want life-sustaining treatment continued should be informed that this is a reasonable decision, but only if it is understood on their part as a request for a continued trial of intervention to determine whether such treatment is reasonably expected to benefit their child.[20] The physician should explain that the decision to continue such treatment is not irreversible. Indeed, the physician should advise parents that he or she will make recommendations about continuing or discontinuing the trial of intervention. Whether continuing life-sustaining treatment is medically reasonable is a professional, expert medical judgment, not a lay judgment. It is essential that this aspect of decision making be made clear to parents who request that "everything be done" to save their child.

"Quality of life" is a phrase often used in perinatal ethics but without a clear understanding of its meaning. The phrase comes from the social sciences and means engaging in valued life tasks and deriving satisfaction from doing so. While infants surely display distinctive personalities and have developmental tasks, they do not have the developmental capacity to conceive of valued life tasks, much less to derive satisfaction from their pursuit over many months and years. As we pointed out in Chapter 1, the concept of quality of life, therefore, does not have clinical application in perinatal ethics. Limiting life-sustaining neonatal critical care based on quality of life considerations is, therefore, not ethically permissible.

3.5 Burdens on parents and society

There is no doubt that the parents of survivors with major physical and/or mental impairments find themselves confronted with a life of providing long-term care to their child. Most parents do not anticipate having this kind of relationship with a newborn child. The physical, psychosocial, and financial burdens on parents and other family members of providing such long-term care can become considerable, even overwhelming.

Justice requires that such burdens be distributed fairly in society. These long-term care burdens are not a function of parental choice but of the biologic variability of pregnancy in almost cases. In developed countries, the burdens of long-term care can be shared through comprehensive programs to support parents with considerable long-term care burdens, so that these burdens do not become overwhelming. No society can regard itself to be consistent with the requirements of justice in the absence of such a social policy. It is not consistent with professional medical ethics to let a patient die for any reason other than that the limits of beneficence-based and justice-based obligation to treat have been reached. In the absence of futility, in the various senses described above, letting a patient die to reduce parental burden is inconsistent with professional integrity and is, therefore, ethically impermissible in perinatal medicine.[10]

Schooling, occupational therapy, reasonable accommodations in the workplace for the disabled, and other supports for disabled children, are very expensive. It is simply an abrogation of justice for developed countries around the world to allow handicapped children to die so that society can escape its justice-based obligations. Invoking scarce resources as a justification for limiting medical treatment only invites distrust of parents or compounds the distrust of parents from racial and ethnic groups who have experienced unacceptable disparities in health care and social services.

3.6 Conclusion

The professional responsibility model of perinatal ethics guides the perinatologist in developing deliberative clinical ethical judgment about the initiation of and ethically justified limits on obstetric and neonatal intervention in periviable pregnancies. Such deliberative clinical ethical judgment identifies beneficence-based, autonomy-based, and justice-based considerations that should decision making with pregnant patients about the obstetric management of periviability and with parents about the neonatal management of periviability.

3.7 References

1. American College of Obstetricians and Gynecologists. ACOG Practice Bulletin: Clinical Management Guidelines for Obstetrician-Gynecologists: Number 38, September 2002. Perinatal care at the threshold of viability. Obstet Gynecol 2002;100:617–624.

2. MacDonald H, American Academy of Pediatrics, Committee on the Fetus and Newborn. Perinatal care at the threshold of viability. Pediatrics 2002;110:1024–1027.
3. Higgins RD, Delivoria-Papadopoulos M, Raju TNK. Executive summary of the workshop on the border of viability. Pediatrics 2005;115:1392–1396.
4. Skupski DW, Greenough A, Donn SM, Arabin B, Bancalari E, Vladareanu R. Delivery mode for the extremely premature fetus: a statement of the prematurity working group of the World Association of Perinatal Medicine. J Perinat Med 2009;37:583–586.
5. Chervenak FA, McCullough LB. The limits of viability. J Perinat Med 1997;25:418–420.
6. Chervenak FA, McCullough LB, Levene MI. An ethically justified, clinically comprehensive approach to peri-viability: gynaecologic, obstetric, perinatal, and neonatal dimensions. J Obstet Gynaecol 2007;27:3–7.
7. Levene M. Is intensive care for very immature babies justified? Acta Paediatr 2004;92:1–4.
8. Hintz SR, Kendrick DE, Vohr BR, Poole WK, Higgins RD. Changes in neurodevelopmental outcomes at 18 to 22 months' corrected age among infants of less than 25 weeks' gestational age born in 1993–1999. Pediatrics 2005;115:1645–1651.
9. Doyle LW and the Victorian Infant Collaborative Study Group. Neonatal intensive care at borderline viability – is it worth it? Early Human Development 2004;80:103–113.
10. Chervenak FA, McCullough LB, Campbell S. Third trimester abortion: is compassion enough? Br J Obstet Gynaecol 1999;106:293–296.
11. Stoll BJ, Jansen NI, Bell EF, Shankaran AR, et al., for the Eunice Kennedy Shriver National Institute of Child Health and Human Development Neonatal Research Netword. Neonatal outcomes of extremely premature infants from the NICHD Neonatal Research Network. Pediatrics 2010;126:443–456.
12. Lucey JF, Rowan CA, Shiono P, Wilkinson AR, et al. Fetal infants: the fate of 4172 infants with birth weights of 401 to 500 grams – the Vermont Oxford Network experience (1996–2000). Pediatrics 2004;113:1559–1566.
13. Chervenak FA, Skupski DW, Romero R, Myers MK, Smith-Levitin M, Rosenwaks Z, Thaler HT. How accurate is fetal biometry in the assessment of fetal age? Am J Obstet Gynecol 1998; 178:678–687.
14. Tyson JE, Parikh NA, Langer J, Green C, Higgins RD for the NICHD. Intensive care for extreme prematurity—moving beyond gestational age. N Engl J Med 2008;358:1672–81.
15. Skupski DW, McCullough LB, Levene M, Chervenak FA. Improving Obstetric Estimation of Outcomes of Extremely Premature Neonates: An Evolving Challenge. J Perinat Med 2010;38:19–22.
16. American Heart Association in collaboration with the International Liaison Committee on Resuscitation (IL-COR). Guidelines 2000 for cardiopulmonary resuscitation and emergency cardiovascular care. An international consensus on science. Circulation 2000;102(Suppl. I):I-1–I-384.(a)
17. American Heart Association in collaboration with the International Liaison Committee on Resuscitation (IL-COR). Guidelines 2000 for cardiopulmonary resuscitation and emergency cardiovascular care – an international consensus on science. Resuscitation 2000;46:1–447.(b)
18. Jones JW, McCullough LB. Postoperative futility: a clinical algorithm for setting limits. Br J Surg 2001;88:1153–1154.
19. McCormick RA. To save or let die: the dilemma of modern medicine. JAMA 1974;229:172–176.
20. McGraw MP, Jeffrey Perlman J, Chervenak FA, McCullough LB. Clinical Concepts of Futility and Ethically Justified Limits on Neonatal Care: A Case Presentation of an Infant with Apgar Scores of Zero at One, Five, and Ten Minutes. Am J Perinatol 2006;23:159–162.

3.8 Summary points

- Induced abortion is ethically permissible at 22 weeks gestation or before, permissible at 23 weeks gestation, and ethically impermissible at 24 weeks gestation in the absence of serious fetal anomalies.
- At 22 weeks gestation, there is no ethical obligation to offer or perform aggressive obstetric management or resuscitation, followed by neonatal critical care.
- At 23 weeks, there is no ethical obligation to offer aggressive obstetric and neonatal management, although it is ethically permissible to offer aggressive obstetric management, followed by neonatal resuscitation and critical care as trials of intervention.
- At 24 weeks, in the absence of serious fetal anomalies, it is ethically obligatory to recommend aggressive obstetric management, when it is reliably expected to improve outcomes, followed by neonatal resuscitation and critical care as trials of intervention.
- It is ethically justified to end the trial of neonatal critical care when the patient has a terminal or irreversible condition, as defined in applicable advance directives legislation, or when either physiologic, imminent demise, or clinical or overall futility apply. (See Chapter 7)

4 Intrapartum management

4.1 Introduction

There are many difficult ethical challenges about intrapartum management of pregnancy. We first address the important and often neglected topic of a preventive ethics approach to cesarean delivery. Second, we address recommendations for mode of delivery.[1] Traditional thinking about mode of delivery has been binomial: A cesarean delivery is indicated or not. This traditional thinking obscures clinical circumstances in which offering both cesarean delivery and vaginal is ethically justified.[2] Deliberative clinical ethical judgment about the mode of delivery therefore should consider recommending cesarean delivery, offering both cesarean and vaginal delivery, and recommending vaginal delivery, including the related ethical challenge of how to respond professionally to a request from a pregnant woman for a non-indicated cesarean delivery. We then address the role of destructive procedures in professionally responsible intrapartum management.[3] We close by addressing non-aggressive obstetric management.[4–5]

4.2 A preventive ethics approach to cesarean delivery

Salmeen and Brincat made a valuable contribution to perinatal ethics by documenting the importance of time constraints for informed consent for cesarean delivery. This retrospective study of the range of consent time for cesarean delivery during labor showed that the median time from consent to incision was 48 minutes. For women who underwent cesarean delivery for fetal heart rate indications, the odds of delivering in less than 30 minutes after consent were increased by 4.7. Salmeen and Brincat reasonably conclude that the consent time for cesarean delivery during labor is brief.[6] Given the distractions of labor, and the momentum for surgical intervention that builds as maternal or fetal indications justifiably come to dominate deliberative clinical judgment, obtaining informed consent during labor for cesarean delivery is, by its very nature, ethically challenging.

The best way to address this ethical challenge is with preventive ethics, a concept that we introduced in 1990.[7,8] As explained in Chapter 1, preventive ethics uses the informed consent process to anticipate, prevent, and responsibly manage the potential for ethical conflict between the pregnant woman and her perinatologist. The absence of a preventive ethics approach to decision making with patients about cesarean delivery unwittingly fosters the misperception of the "perfect baby"[9] and misses important opportunities to prepare the pregnant woman for rush of decision making about cesarean delivery documented by Salmeen and Brincat, so that it does not overwhelm her autonomy or birth experience.

The goal of a preventive ethics approach to informed consent for cesarean delivery is to empower the pregnant woman with information about cesarean delivery that she may need later. Given time and adequate support, pregnant women demonstrate the capacity to make informed, scientifically sophisticated decisions about their medical care, e.g. the use of invasive prenatal diagnosis on the basis of the results of non-invasive risk assessment to make decisions about invasive diagnosis in advance of the potential need for it.[10]

An adequately informed consent process for cesarean delivery takes time. This process, by its very nature, requires the pregnant woman to give her attention to her perinatologist, listen carefully, think through and carefully assess the benefits and risks of cesarean delivery, and appreciate that, for maternal or fetal indications, cesarean delivery can become the only medically reasonable alternative for delivery and will therefore be recommended. All of this takes time and a minimum of distraction, which are difficult to achieve under the time constraints that Salmeen and Brincat have documented. Perinatologists should take advantage of the fact that most pregnant women are seen prenatally, some even preconception, creating multiple opportunities for an effective preventive ethics approach to informed consent for cesarean delivery.

As part of routine prenatal care, every pregnant woman should be informed that cesarean delivery occurs in about one third of pregnancies.[11] Every pregnant woman should also appreciate that a low-risk pregnancy can change rapidly into a high-risk pregnancy during the intrapartum period and that cesarean delivery may become necessary for either maternal or fetal indications. The perinatologist should elicit the patient's attitudes about cesarean delivery and tailor subsequent information accordingly.

For some women, depending on their medical condition and informational needs, decisions about cesarean delivery require more than this general information that every pregnant women should receive. For these women, the perinatologist should explain that cesarean delivery is not always dichotomous.[2] The perinatologist may need to identify for the pregnant woman the medically reasonable alternatives for the intrapartum management of her pregnancy, i.e. those reliably expected to result in net clinical benefit to the pregnant, fetal, or neonatal patient. The perinatologist should explain that in such circumstances, which we address in greater detail below, cesarean delivery may be recommended.

A preventive ethics approach to the informed consent process for cesarean delivery should become an accepted component of routine perinatal care. Taking a preventive ethics approach to the informed consent process for cesarean delivery should be expected to enhance the autonomy of pregnant women, by preparing them to cope more effectively with the complexity and urgency of decision making about cesarean delivery during the intrapartum period. A preventive ethics approach creates the opportunity to identify and resolve potential conflicts about cesarean delivery.[2]

4.3 Recommendations regarding mode of delivery

4.3.1 Recommending cesarean delivery

Sometimes, cesarean delivery is well supported and vaginal delivery is not supported in beneficence-based deliberative clinical judgment. For example, when there is a previous classical incision on the uterus, cesarean delivery is clearly preferable to vaginal delivery because cesarean delivery prevents the fetal and maternal risk of a ruptured classical incision in the uterus in up to 12% of cases.[12] Vaginal delivery, in these circumstances, would result in a substantial increase in maternal–fetal morbidity and mortality. Because vaginal delivery involves unnecessary and preventable harms and cesarean delivery prevents these harms, no well-founded beneficence-based clinical judgment could support offering vaginal delivery to women with a previous classical uterine incision. The professional responsibility model of perinatal ethics, therefore, requires that only cesarean delivery should be offered and recommended to such patients. With the patient's consent, it should then be performed.

4.3.2 Offering both cesarean delivery and vaginal delivery

Sometimes, cesarean delivery and vaginal delivery are both well supported in beneficence-based deliberative clinical judgment. In some clinical circumstances, there is scientific controversy as to whether cesarean delivery or vaginal delivery is the better alternative. Competing well-founded, beneficence-based, deliberative clinical judgments regarding how to balance the fetal benefit of preventing harm against the maternal risk of cesarean delivery generate these controversies. Whenever two management strategies are well supported in beneficence-based, deliberative clinical judgment, the professional responsibility model requires that both should be offered to the pregnant woman so that she can exercise her autonomy meaningfully. Such disclosure empowers the woman to emphasize her own perspective in balancing maternal and fetal risks. Not offering all management options well supported in beneficence-based clinical judgment restricts and does not empower the exercise of her autonomy by the pregnant woman and is, therefore, professionally irresponsible. Professional responsibility requires offering both cesarean and vaginal delivery and then performing either cesarean or vaginal delivery, based on the pregnant woman's informed consent.

Trial of labor after a low transverse cesarean delivery (TOLAC), or vaginal birth after cesarean delivery (VBAC), illustrates this category. In 2010 both and United States National Institutes of Health (NIH) Consensus Panel[13] and American College of Obstetricians and Gynecologists (ACOG)[14] issued updated statements on vaginal birth after caesarean delivery (VBAC). In the United Kingdom, the National Institute for Health and Clinical Excellence (NICE) report provides a thorough review of the clinical benefits and risks to both pregnant and fetal patients and calls for an evidence-based approach to the informed consent process.[15] Both agree that there should be a thorough, evidence-based informed consent process, in which pregnant women with a prior caesarean delivery be counseled concerning VBAC. Here we provide an ethically justified, practical to the informed consent process for TOLAC.

When both repeat caesarean and TOLAC are supported in evidence-based, beneficence-based, deliberative clinical judgment, both should be offered in clinical settings where TOLAC can be performed safely. The NIH Consensus Panel[13] and ACOG[14] statements are in consensus that TOLAC after a previous single low transverse uterine incision is medically reasonable and should be offered when there has been one previous low transverse incision. In the professional responsibility model of perinatal ethics, the evidence supports the beneficence-based clinical judgment that the clinical risks of TOLAC, to both pregnant and fetal patients, are acceptable when there has been one previous low transverse incision. Planned repeat caesarean delivery also has acceptable risks to both pregnant and fetal patients. Both, therefore, should be offered in the informed consent process to the pregnant woman with one previous low transverse incision, because both are medically reasonable in this clinical circumstance. Counseling about these alternatives should be non-directive.

Controversy exists about TOLAC after two low transverse incisions. The ACOG statement, on the basis of Level B evidence, states: "Women with two previous low transverse incisions may be considered candidates for TOLAC."[14] The NIH Consensus Panel was silent on this topic.[13] Level B evidence is inherently controversial in beneficence-based clinical judgment. As a result, perinatologists should responsibly manage competing evidence-based, beneficence clinical judgment about the safety for pregnant and fetal patients of TOLAC when the pregnant woman has had two previous low transverse incisions. In the informed consent process, responsible management is achieved by offering TOLAC, but only when the perinatologist explains the uncertainties of the current state of the evidence in this clinical circumstance.

The professional responsibility model of perinatal ethics provides the basis for an ethically justified, practical approach to of offering TOLAC in the informed consent process with pregnant women with a prior caesarean delivery. For women with one previous low transverse incision, both TOLAC and planned repeat caesarean delivery should be offered. TOLAC should only be offered in clinical settings properly equipped and staffed to do so. Perinatologists should recommend against TOLAC when the pregnant woman has had a previous classical incision. TOLAC after two previous low transverse incisions may be offered, provided that the informed consent process presents the uncertainties of the evidence.

4.3.3 Recommending vaginal delivery

Sometimes vaginal delivery is well supported in beneficence-based clinical judgment and cesarean delivery is not supported in beneficence-based deliberative clinical judgment. When deliberative beneficence-based clinical judgment concludes that vaginal delivery is the only medically reasonable alternative, it should be recommended. Cesarean delivery involves a clinically significant increased risk of unnecessary and preventable maternal morbidity and mortality.[16] The unnecessary and preventable nature of the risks of cesarean delivery loom large in this beneficence-based deliberative clinical judgment. As a consequence, the professional responsibility model prohibits the offering of cesarean delivery; only vaginal delivery should be recommended.

This three-part, rather than binomial, approach to responsibly managing the ethical challenges of mode of delivery underscores the centrality of the professional integrity in the professional responsibility model of perinatal ethics, and therefore in the informed-consent process. In some clinical situations, such as a previous low transverse uterine incision, there are advantages of elective repeat cesarean delivery for the physician, including time saved, convenience, and possibly increased remuneration. It is a clear and unacceptable violation of the professional integrity of the physician's role in the informed consent process for the physician to distort this process in pursuit of such advantages.[17]

4.3.4 Responding to requests for non-indicated cesarean delivery

Some women will, unprompted, request non-indicated cesarean delivery. This is known as patient-choice caesarean delivery, maternal-choice caesarean delivery, or cesarean delivery on demand. One review reported a range from 2 % of primary cesarean deliveries in Canada to 17 % in Australia and perhaps as high as 80 % in Brazil.[18]

How to respond to such requests has become controversial throughout the world. In the United States, for example, the American College of Obstetricians and Gynecologists (ACOG) stated in a committee opinion in 2003 that, while the right of patients to refuse unwanted surgery is well known, less clear is the right of patients to have a surgical procedure when scientific evidence supporting it is incomplete, of poor quality, or totally lacking.[19] The Committee concluded that the evidence to support the benefit of caesarean delivery is still incomplete and that there are insufficient morbidity and mortality data to compare caesarean delivery with planned vaginal delivery. In addition, the United States National Institutes of Health (NIH) convened a 2006 conference regarding this issue that concluded that there is insufficient evidence to evaluate fully the benefits and risks of primary caesarean delivery as compared to vaginal delivery, and that more research is needed.[20] The NIH conference concluded: "The magnitude of caesarean delivery on maternal request is difficult to quantify. There is insufficient evidence to evaluate fully the benefits and risks of caesarean delivery on maternal request compared with planned vaginal delivery. Any decision to perform a caesarean delivery on maternal request should be carefully individualized and consistent with ethical principles."[20]

In the United Kingdom, the NICE 2011 report notes the increasing rates of "maternal request for caesarean delivery" and that a common reason for such requests is the pregnant woman's concern for the safety of her baby. The report also notes that obstetricians implement as much as half of the requests that they receive. The report provides guidance for obstetricians in response to maternal request for caesarean delivery: "When a woman requests a CS the first response should be to determine the reason for the request and the factors that are contributing to the request. This can then be followed by the provision of information that compares the risks and benefits of planned CS and vaginal birth."[15] The report makes the following recommendation: "For women requesting a CS, if after discussion and offer of support (including perinatal mental health support for women with anxiety about childbirth), a vaginal birth is still not an acceptable option, offer a planned CS."[7] Obstetricians unwilling to perform caesarean delivery on maternal request "should refer the woman to an obstetrician who will perform CS."[15]

These influential statements and reports emphasize clinical benefits and risks and the communication of this clinical information in the informed consent process. Put another way, ethics is an essential, though often implicit, component of patient-choice caesarean delivery.[21,22] Here we provide an explicitly ethically justified, practical guidance for perinatologists in response the patient-choice caesarean delivery based on the professional responsibility model of perinatal ethics.

Caesarean delivery has become safer over time, with the advancement in surgical techniques, anesthetic options, antimicrobial availability, and blood banking techniques. There are several potential maternal and fetal benefits of undergoing caesarean delivery versus planned vaginal delivery. Comprehensive beneficence-based clinical judgment requires that the potential benefits of caesarean delivery be balanced against the benefits of planned vaginal delivery and the risks of caesarean delivery.

Currently, beneficence-based clinical judgment favors vaginal delivery.[2] Hence, counseling should be directive, as opposed to non-directive counseling, in response to requests for non-indicated cesarean delivery: the perinatologist should clearly recommend vaginal delivery. We, therefore, disagree with the NICE report's purely non-directive approach.[15]

Respect for autonomy remains the rationale for promotion of caesarean delivery. Respect for autonomy surely is a core ethical obligation. Only in maternal-rights-based reductionism does it create an absolute obligation, i.e. an obligation that admits of no exceptions. The professional responsibility model rejects this account, as explained in Chapter 1. Instead, autonomy-based obligations must in all cases be balanced against beneficence-based obligations to both the pregnant and fetal patients. A perinatologist should not conclude that every request for a caesarean delivery should be implemented routinely; patients' requests do not identify the medically reasonable alternatives for patient, deliberative clinical ethical judgment does.[23,24]

Respect for autonomy is implemented by adherence to the informed consent process, as described in Chapter 1. The perinatologist is expected to exercise professional, beneficence-based clinical judgment when making clinical recommendations, and present the medically reasonable alternatives as well as the alternative of nonintervention. The patient can then exercise her rights to accept or refuse intervention. Respect for autonomy in the informed consent does not warrant routine offering of caesarean delivery, because doing so is not supported in beneficence-based clinical judgment. Routinely offering cesarean delivery does not empower pregnant women.

Considering beneficence-based and autonomy-based obligations to the pregnant woman together, there is no ethical obligation to offer non-indicated caesarean delivery to all pregnant women. Offering caesarean delivery to all patients does not promote their health-related interests. Perinatologists must rigorously adhere to the requirements of professional integrity, to prevent potential bias from influencing the physician's discussion with the patient introduced by economic gain or other forms of self-interest. The NICE report's indications for offering planned caesarean delivery do not include routine offering of caesarean delivery,[7] and therefore reflect this ethical position.

It is very important not to misinterpret the ethical principle of respect for patient autonomy. The physician's medical expertise and authority should not be marshaled to convince a patient to choose caesarean delivery. Respect for patients' autonomy should not be used as an excuse to persuade more women to undergo caesarean delivery for reasons such as the physician's convenience or desire to reduce professional liability. When patients request caesarean delivery, perinatologists-in their capacity as patients' advocates for clinical management supported by deliberative clinical judgment-must guide patients through the labyrinth of medical information toward a decision that respects both the patient's autonomy and the physician's obligation to optimize maternal-fetal health. Providing evidence-based information about the clinical benefits and risks of non-indicated caesarean delivery, as called for in the NICE report,[15] meets this important autonomy-enhancing goal.

We can now answer a question that Feldman and Freiman[25] asked many years ago: "If an informed patient opts for prophylactic cesarean section at term, can it be denied?" If such a request is well supported in autonomy-based clinical judgment, which will be rare, it should be carried out by the physician, or an appropriate referral should be made. Feldman and Freiman also suggested that patients should be informed of the "very real risks associated with the passive anticipation of vaginal delivery after fetal maturity has been reached."[25] However, we conclude that this obligation does not exist because an affirmative answer makes the incorrect assumption that cesarean delivery is supported in beneficence-based clinical judgment.

Well-supported requests for cesarean delivery contrast with those that are not well supported in autonomy-based clinical judgment (i.e. when the goals expressed in the patient's preference for cesarean delivery can be achieved without delivering by cesarean section). For example, a woman who is in pain during labor may request cesarean delivery for relief of the pain. However, this goal can be achieved by administration of analgesia, whereas cesarean delivery for pain relief will result in more pain and unnecessary risk of morbidity and mortality. The preference is internally inconsistent, and therefore not well supported in autonomy-based clinical judgment. When a pregnant woman's request for non-indicated cesarean delivery is not well supported in deliberative clinical judgment, the perinatologist should recommend strongly against cesarean delivery and should strongly recommend vaginal delivery.

4.4 The role of destructive procedures

4.4.1 Cephalocentesis for intrapartum management of hydrocephalus

Cephalocentesis involves the drainage of an enlarged fetal head, secondary to hydrocephalus.[26] Fetal hydrocephalus is caused by obstruction of cerebrospinal flow and is diagnosed by such sonographic signs as dilatation of the atrium or body of the lateral ventricles.[27] In the third trimester, macrocephaly often accompanies the ventriculomegaly. In addition, sonography can diagnose hydrocephalus in association with gross abnormalities suggestive of poor prognosis, for example, hydranencephaly, microcephaly, encephalocele, alobar holoprosencephaly, or thanatophoric dysplasia with cloverleaf skull.[27] In the absence of defined anatomical abnormalities, however, diagnostic imaging is, at the present time, unable to predict the outcome. Although cortical mantle thickness can be measured with ultrasound, its value as a prognostic index is not established.[28]

Cephalocentesis should be performed under simultaneous ultrasound guidance so that needle placement into the cerebrospinal fluid is facilitated. An 18-gauge needle is used with subsequent collapse of the cranial bones, the endpoint for this procedure. Enough fluid is drained to permit reduction of the skull diameters so that passage through the birth canal is possible.[27] Cephalocentesis is a potentially destructive procedure. Perinatal death following cephalocentesis has been reported in over 90 % of cases.[26] The sonographic visualization of intracranial bleeding during cephalocentesis, and the demonstration of this hemorrhage at autopsy, further emphasize the morbid nature of the procedure. However, if decompression is performed in a controlled manner, the mortality may be reduced.

4.4.2 Isolated fetal hydrocephalus

There is considerable potential for normal, sometimes superior, intellectual function for fetuses with even extreme, isolated hydrocephalus.[29–32] However, as a group, infants with isolated hydrocephalus experience a greater incidence of intellectual disability and early death than the general population. In addition, associated anomalies may go undetected, and a fetus may be incorrectly diagnosed as having isolated hydrocephalus.[28] One thing is clear in obstetric ethics: A viable at-term fetus with isolated hydrocephalus is a fetal patient.

There are compelling, beneficence-based ethical reasons for concluding that continuing existence of fetuses with isolated hydrocephalus is in their interest. Beneficence directs the physician to prevent mortality and morbidity for the fetal patient. Beneficence also directs the physician to undertake interventions that ameliorate conditions such as intellectual disability. The probability of intellectual disability does not diminish the interests of the fetal patient with isolated hydrocephalus in continuing existence because (1) it is impossible to predict which fetuses with isolated hydrocephalus will have intellectual disability, and (2) the degree of such disability cannot be predicted in advance.

The beneficence-based obligation of the physician caring for the fetus with macrocephaly is to recommend strongly and to attain the woman's consent to perform a cesarean delivery because this clinical intervention clearly involves the least risk of mortality, morbidity, and disability for the fetus compared with cephalocentesis to permit subsequent vaginal delivery. Even when performed under maximal therapeutic conditions (i.e. under sonographic guidance), cephalocentesis cannot reasonably be regarded as protecting or promoting the health-related interests of the fetal patient with isolated hydrocephalus with macrocephaly. This procedure is followed by a high rate of perinatal mortality, fetal heart rate deceleration, and pathologic evidence of intracranial bleeding.[26] Cephalocentesis, therefore, cannot reasonably be construed as an ethically justifiable mode of management, insofar as it is inconsistent with beneficence-based obligations to avoid increased mortality and morbidity risks for the fetal patient. Cephalocentesis, employed with a destructive intent, is altogether antithetical to the beneficence-based prohibition against killing.[17]

It is essential in perinatal ethics that beneficence-based obligations to the fetal patient be balanced against beneficence-based and autonomy-based obligations to the pregnant woman. First, the physician has a beneficence-based obligation to avoid performing a cesarean delivery because the possibility of morbidity and mortality for the woman is higher than that associated with vaginal delivery. Respect for autonomy obligates the physician to undertake only those interventions or forms of treatment to which the woman has given voluntary, informed consent. Informed consent is grounded in an autonomy-based right of the pregnant woman to control what happens to her body. In particular, the woman has the right to authorize or refuse operative intervention – those that are, as well as those that are not, consistent with the physician's beneficence-based obligations.[17]

The above analysis sets the stage for considering the full complexity of the management of the fetal patient with isolated hydrocephalus with macrocephaly: Beneficence-based and autonomy-based obligations to the pregnant woman, as well as beneficence-based obligations to her fetus, must all be considered for clinical ethical judgment to be complete, and therefore reliable. If, with informed consent, the woman authorizes cesarean delivery, there is no conflict among these obligations.

By contrast, her physician faces a significant and challenging ethical conflict if the woman refuses cesarean delivery. This conflict should be resolved in favor of the beneficence-based obligations to the fetal patient, because the harm to the fetal patient is final, namely, death, and will occur with high probability. Moreover, if the fetal patient survives (death is not guaranteed by cephalocentesis), it is likely to be more damaged due to intracranial hemorrhage than if cesarean delivery is performed. Morbidity and mortality of the pregnant woman are both minimal, and therefore risks that she ought to accept to protect the fetal patient's interest.[17] Such ethical conflict should be prevented by employing the preventive ethics strategies described in Chapter 1.[7]

If these preventive ethics strategies do not succeed and the pregnant woman continues to refuse cesarean delivery, the physician confronts tragic circumstances. If neither cesarean delivery nor cephalocentesis is performed, the woman is at risk for uterine rupture and death, and the fetal patient is at risk for death. This logic of beneficence-based obligations is to prevent such total and irreversible harm. Therefore, we believe that because of the grave nature of possible consequences for the woman and her fetus, because of the dangers for the woman of performing a surgical procedure on a resistant patient, and because of the pitfalls of attempted legal coercion, the physician should act on beneficence-based obligations to the woman in such an extreme circumstance. The fetal patient is at high risk for death under either alternative. The woman's death, at least, can be avoided. Serious beneficence-based obligations to the fetal patient on the part of both the physician and the pregnant woman will probably be violated and a needless death will most probably result, however, by performing a cephalocentesis. Herein lies the tragedy of these circumstances. To avoid this tragedy, redoubled efforts of preventive ethics should be undertaken. Carefully explaining the fact that cephalocentesis does not guarantee death and may produce a worse outcome is very powerfully persuasive. In those rare cases in which this effort at respectful persuasion fails, cephalocentesis should be performed in the least destructive way possible.

4.4.3 Hydrocephalus with severe associated abnormalities

Some abnormalities that occur in association with fetal hydrocephalus are severe in nature for the child afflicted with them. We define "severe" abnormalities as those that either are (1) incompatible with continued existence, e.g. bilateral renal agenesis or thanatophoric dysplasia with cloverleaf skull, or (2) compatible with survival in some cases but result in virtual absence of cognitive function, e.g. trisomy 18 or alobar holoprosencephaly.[33] Because there is no available intervention to prevent postnatal death in the first group, beneficence-based obligations of the physician and the pregnant woman to attempt to prolong the life of the fetal patient are nonexistent. No ethical theory and no version of obstetric ethics based on beneficence and respect for autonomy obligate the physician to attempt the impossible. For the second group, beneficence-based obligations of the physician and the pregnant woman to sustain the life of the fetal patient are minimal because the disability imposed by the abnormality is severe. In these cases, the potential for cognitive development, and therefore the achievement of other psychosocial goods for the child, e.g. relationships with others are virtually absent. Such fetuses are fetal patients to which there are owed only minimal beneficence-based obligations.

In these circumstances, the woman is released from her beneficence-based obligations to the at-term fetal patient to place herself at risk, because no significant clinical good can be achieved by cesarean delivery for the fetal patient or the child it will become. There remain only the autonomy-based and beneficence-based obligations of the physician to the pregnant woman. After the preceding analysis of these obligations, we conclude that the physician's overriding moral obligations are to the pregnant woman's voluntary and informed decision about employment of cephalocentesis.

Because there are no weighty beneficence-based obligations to the fetus in such clinical and ethical circumstances, the physician may justifiably recommend a choice between cesarean delivery and cephalocentesis to enable vaginal delivery. There are obvious advantages to the woman's health by the avoidance of cesarean delivery. However, cesarean delivery permits women, who wish to do so, to have a live birth and satisfy religious or other convictions or help with the grieving process. A cesarean delivery performed in this clinical setting is best viewed as an autonomy-based maternal indication. Because the prognosis for infants with hydrocephalus associated with severe anomalies is poor, we believe that intrapartum fetal death resulting from cephalocentesis would not be a tragic outcome in the sense that it would be in the death of a fetal patient with isolated hydrocephalus.

4.4.4 Hydrocephalus with other associated anomalies

On the continuum between the extreme cases of isolated hydrocephalus and hydrocephalus with severe associated abnormalities, there is a variety of cases of hydrocephalus associated with macrocephaly with other abnormalities with varying degrees of impairment of cognitive physical function. They range from hypoplastic distal phalanges to spina bifida to encephalocele.[28] Because these conditions have varying prognoses, it would be clinically inappropriate, and therefore, ethically misleading to treat this third category as homogeneous. Therefore, we propose a working distinction between different kinds of prognoses. The first, we call "probably promising", by which we mean that there is a significant possibility the child will experience cognitive development with learning disabilities and physical disabilities that perhaps can be ameliorated to some extent. The second, we call "probably poor". By this phrase, we mean that there is only a limited possibility for cognitive development because of learning disabilities and physical disabilities that cannot be ameliorated to a significant extent. We propose these definitions as tentative, so they are subject to revision as clinical and ethical investigation of such associated anomalies continues. As a consequence, our ethical analysis of these two categories cannot be carried out as fully as extensively as those in the previous two sections. In essence, we propose that the clinical continuum in these cases is paralleled by an ethical continuum or progressively less weighty, beneficence-based obligations to the fetal patient.

When the prognosis is probably promising, e.g. isolated arachnoid cyst, there are serious beneficence-based obligations to the fetal patient. However, they are not necessarily on the same order as those that occur in cases of isolated hydrocephalus. (It has been suggested that any associated anomaly may increase the possibility of a poor outcome.[27]) Therefore, in such cases with a prognosis of probably promising, we propose that the physician recommend cesarean delivery although perhaps not as vigorously as in cases of isolated hydrocephalus. A pregnant woman's informed refusal of cesarean delivery should therefore be respected.

In cases when the prognosis, even though uncertain, is probably poor, e.g. encephalocele, beneficence-based obligations to the fetal patient are less weighty than those owed to the fetal patient with a promising prognosis. These cases, then, resemble ethically those of hydrocephalus with severe anomalies, with the proviso that some, albeit limited, benefits can be achieved for the fetal patient by cesarean delivery and aggressive perinatal treatment. Nonetheless, the physician may, in these cases, justifiably accept an informed voluntary decision by the woman for cephalocentesis followed by vaginal delivery. However, the physician cannot assume an advocacy role for such a decision with the same level of ethical confidence that he or she can in cases of hydrocephalus associated with severe anomalies.

4.5 Non-aggressive obstetric management

As explained in Chapter 1, in the professional responsibility model of perinatal ethics, when the pregnant woman presents for clinical care, the viable fetus becomes a patient. Before viability, the fetus becomes a patient when the pregnant woman confers this moral status on it. When the fetus is a patient, both the perinatologist and the pregnant woman have beneficence-based obligations to protect and life and health of the fetal patient, subject to the constraint that the pregnant woman is obligated to take only reasonable risks to her life and health to benefit the fetal and neonatal patient.[17] Aggressive management is the ethical standard of care for pregnancies going to term, i.e. in which the pregnant has conferred the moral status of being a patient on the previable fetus or in which the fetus has become viable.

4.5.1 Aggressive and non-aggressive obstetric management defined

By aggressive management, we mean optimizing perinatal outcome by utilizing effective antepartum and intrapartum diagnostic and therapeutic modalities, such as fetal monitoring, ultrasound surveillance, cesarean delivery, and delivery in a tertiary center. By non-aggressive management, we mean that these modalities are not used and all indications for clinical intervention are maternal. Non-aggressive management should be distinguished from feticide, which is the direct killing of the in utero fetus. We address the ethics of feticide elsewhere in this book (See Chapter 2), where we identify circumstances in which feticide is ethically justified and circumstances in which it is not ethically justified.

Non-aggressive management is justifiably offered when a decision has been made not to intervene in a pregnancy with the expectation that the fetus will die. These decisions can be made after viability, but also before viability when a fetal anomaly has been detected and the woman does not elect to terminate her pregnancy for religious or other reasons. The ethical concept of the fetus as a patient has implications for when this decision can be made and implemented with ethical justification.

The major clinical implication of the ethical concept of the fetus as a patient is that the burden of proof is on the perinatologist to justify non-aggressive fetal management, because it is otherwise not consistent with the beneficence-based obligation to protect the life and health of the fetal patient. This burden of proof is met when the beneficence-based obligations to the fetal patient to preserve its life cease to exist or have become minimal.

4.5.2 When beneficence-based obligations to the fetal patient cease to exist

Beneficence-based obligations to the fetal patient to preserve its life cease to exist when there is (1) a very high probability, but sometimes less than complete certainty, about the diagnosis and, (2) a very high probability of death as an outcome of the anomaly diagnosed.[34,35] Diagnoses, to which the two clinical ethical criteria for no beneficence-based obligation to preserve fetal life apply, include anencephaly, triploidy, and bilateral renal agenesis.

4.5.3 When beneficence-based obligations to the fetal patient become minimal

Beneficence-based obligations to the fetal patient to preserve its life become minimal when there is (1) a very high probability, but sometimes less than complete certainty, about the diagnosis and, (2) survival with a very high probability of severe and irreversible deficit of cognitive developmental capacity as a result of the anomaly diagnosed.[34,35] Diagnoses to which the two criteria for a minimal beneficence-based obligation to preserve fetal life apply include trisomy 13, trisomy 18 that result in the severe and irreversible absence of cognitive and developmental capacity, and alobar holoprosencephaly.

We emphasize that there are fetal anomalies to which neither set of criteria apply. These include Down Syndrome and achondroplasia. For these fetuses, the beneficence-based obligation to preserve the life and health of the fetal patient remains intact throughout pregnancy and justifies aggressive for fetal indications and non-aggressive management is not ethically permissible.

When the two criteria for there being no longer a beneficence-based obligation to preserve fetal life apply, it is appropriate to regard the fetus as a dying patient, for whom non-aggressive management is ethically justified. This conclusion reflects the now widely accepted beneficence-based ethical standard of care that non-aggressive management of life-threatening events is appropriate for the clinical care of dying patients. When the two criteria for a minimal beneficence-based obligation to preserve the life of the fetal patient apply, it is appropriate in beneficence-based to regard aggressive management as imposing iatrogenic and disease-related burdens on the fetal patient that will not alter the outcome. There is no beneficence-based obligation to attempt the impossible, especially when the iatrogenic burden of such an attempt is considerable.

4.5.4 Counseling the pregnant woman in the informed consent process for non-aggressive obstetric management

These clinical ethical implications of the ethical concept of the fetus as a patient for non-aggressive fetal management have important implications for how the pregnant woman should be counseled during the informed consent process, when either set of clinical ethical criteria are met. In all cases, the pregnant woman should be provided with a clear account of the nature and prognosis of the fetus' anomaly/ies, the degree of certainty of diagnosis, and its outcome, especially severe and irreversible loss of cognitive developmental capacity. The perinatologist should make a reasonable effort to ensure that she understands this information, in the context of maximal psychosocial support from her spouse or partner, family members, and others, as she selects. The perinatologist should make clear to these individuals that the ultimate decision belongs to the pregnant woman and their role is to be supportive and respectful of her.

The next step is to offer her a choice between non-aggressive and aggressive fetal management. We take this position because some women will want to have the opportunity to try to have their child born alive, for a wide variety of reasons, including helping with the grieving process. Counseling about this choice should be non-directive. The physician should endeavor not to express or imply an acceptable choice on the part of the pregnant woman. These are complicated matters for the pregnant woman to consider, and therefore a physician should be present to provide clinical management and direction. The physician has the preventive ethics obligation to inform neonatology of the plan for non-aggressive obstetric management.

4.6 Conclusion

Perhaps more than for any other aspect of perinatal medicine, ethics is an essential component of intrapartum management. To manage pregnant patients without an understanding of the ethics of intrapartum management is inadequate and inappropriate. The professional responsibility model of perinatal ethics provides the antidote, because it guides the perinatologist and pregnant woman in decision making about intrapartum management. The decision-making process should based on the recognition that decision making is not binomial. A preventive ethics approach should be initiated and then followed with the informed consent process for intrapartum management, including mode of delivery and, when ethically justified, destructive procedures and non-aggressive obstetric management.

4.7 References

1. Chervenak FA, McCullough LB. An ethically justified algorithm for offering, recommending, and performing cesarean delivery and its application in managed care practice. Obstet Gynecol 1995;87:302–305.
2. Kalish RB, McCullough LB, Chervenak FA. Decision-making about caesarean delivery. Lancet 2006;367:883–45.
3. Chasen S, Chervenak FA, McCullough LB. The role of cephalocentesis in modern obstetrics. Am J Obstet Gynecol 2001;185:734–736.
4. Chervenak FA, McCullough LB. Non-aggressive obstetric management: an option for some fetal anomalies during the third trimester. JAMA 1989;261:3439–3440.
5. Chervenak FA, McCullough LB. Ethical dimensions of non-aggressive fetal management. Semin Fetal Neonatal Med 2008;13:316–319.
6. Salmeen K, Brincat C. Time from consent to cesarean delivery during labor. Am J Obstet Gynecol 2013;209:212.e1–6.
7. Chervenak FA, McCullough LB. Clinical guides to preventing ethical conflicts between pregnant women and their physicians. Am J Obstet Gynecol 1990;162:303–307.
8. Chervenak FA, McCullough LB. Preventive ethics for cesarean delivery: the time has come. Am J Obstet Gynecol 2013;209:166–167.
9. Chervenak FA, McCullough LB, Brent RL. The perils of the imperfect expectation of the perfect baby. Am J Obstet Gynecol 2010;203:101.e1–5.

10. Nicolaides KH, Chervenak FA, McCullough LB, et al. Evidence-based obstetric ethics and informed decision-making about invasive diagnosis after first-trimester assessment for risk of trisomy 21. Am J Obstet Gynecol 2005;193:322–326.
11. Hamilton BE, Ventura SJ, Osterman MJK, Wilson EC, Mathews TJ. Births: final data for 2010. U. S. Department of Health and Human Services. Centers for Disease Control and Prevention. National Vital Statistics Report. August 28, 2012;61(1):1–72. Available at www.cdc.gov/nchs/data/nvsr/nvsr61/nvsr61_01.pdf, accessed March 8, 2014.
12. American College of Obstetricians and Gynecologists, Committee on Obstetric Practice. Vaginal delivery after a previous cesarean birth. ACOG committee opinion no. 143. Washington, DC: American College of Obstetricians and Gynecologists, 1994.
13. National Institutes of Health. National Institutes of Health Consensus Development Conference Statement vaginal birth after cesarean: new insights March 8–10, 2010. Semin Perinatal 2010;34:351–365.
14. American College of Obstetricians and Gynecologists. ACOG Practice bulletin no. 115: vaginal birth after prior cesarean delivery. Obstet Gynecol 2010;116(2 Pt 1):450–463.
15. Caesarean Section: National institute of Health and Clinical Excellence Guideline; 2nd ed. London, UK: RCOG, 2011.
16. American College of Obstetricians and Gynecologists and Society for Maternal-Fetal Medicine. Obstetric care consensus: safe prevention of the primary cesarean delivery. Number 1 March 2014. Available at www.acog.org/Resources_And_Publications/Obstetric_Care_Consensus_Series/Safe_Prevention_of_the_Primary_Cesarean_Delivery, accessed March 8, 2014.
17. McCullough LB, Chervenak FA. Ethics in Obstetrics and Gynecology. New York: Oxford University Press, 1994.
18. D'Souza R, Arulkumaran S. To "C" or not to "C" Cesarean delivery upon maternal request: a review of facts, figures and guidelines. J Perinat Med 2013;41:5–15.
19. American College of Obstetrics and Gynecology. ACOG Committee Opinion. Surgery and patient choice: the ethics of decision making. Obstet Gynecol 2003;102:1101–6.
20. [No authors listed]. NIH State-of-the Science Conference Statement on Cesarean Delivery on Maternal Request. NIH Consens State Sci Statements. 2006 Mar 27–29;23(1):1–29.
21. Minkoff H. Powederly KR, Chervenak FA, McCullough LB. Ethical dimensions of elective primary cesarean delivery. Obstet Gynecol 2004;103:387–392.
22. Minkoff H, Chervenak FA. Elective primary cesarean delivery. N Engl J Med 2003;348:946–950.
23. Brett AS, McCullough LB. When patients request specific interventions: Defining the limits of the physician's obligation. N Engl J Med 1986;315:1347–51.
24. Brett AS, McCullough LB. Addressing requests by patients for non-beneficial interventions. JAMA 2012:307:149–50.
25. Feldman GB, Freiman JA. Prophylactic cesarean section at term? N Engl J Med 1985;312:1264–1267.
26. Chervenak FA, Romero R. Is there a role for fetal cephalocentesis in modern obstetrics? Am J Perinatol 1984;1:170–3.
27. Chervenak FA, Isaacson G, Campbell S. Anomalies of the cranium and its contents. Textbook of ultrasound in obstetrics and gynecology. Pp. 825–52. Boston: Little, Brown, 1993.
28. Chervenak FA, Berkowitz RL, Tortora M, et al. Management of fetal hydrocephalus. Am J Obstet Gynecol 1985;151:933–7.
29. Raimondi AJ, Soare P. Intellectual development in shunted hydrocephalic children. Am J Dis Child 1974;127:664.
30. McCullough DC, Balzer-Martin LA. Current prognosis in overt neonatal hydrocephalus. J Neurosurg 1982;57:378.
31. Sutton LN, Bruce DA, Schut L. Hydranencephaly versus maximal hydrocephalus: an important clinical distinction. Neurosurgery 1980;6:35.

32. Lorber J. The results of early treatment on extreme hydrocephalus. Med Child Neurol (Suppl) 1968;16:21.
33. Chervenak FA, McCullough LB. An ethically justified, clinically comprehensive management strategy for third-trimester pregnancies complicated by fetal anomalies. Obstet Gynecol 1990;75:311–6.
34. Chervenak FA, McCullough LB, Campbell S. Is third trimester abortion justified? Brit J Obstet Gynaecol. 1995;102:434–435.
35. Chervenak FA, McCullough LB, Campbell S. Third trimester abortion: Is compassion enough? Brit J Obstet Gynæcol 1999;106:293–296.

4.8 Summary Points

- Decision making about intrapartum management is not binomial.
- Perinatologists should routinely adopt a preventive ethics approach to intrapartum management.
- For women with one previous low transverse incision, the perinatologist should offer both trial of labor after cesarean delivery (TOLAC) and planned repeat caesarean delivery. The perinatologist should offer TOLAC only in clinical settings properly equipped and staffed to do so.
- Perinatologists should recommend against TOLAC when the pregnant woman has had a previous classical incision.
- Perinatologists may offer TOLAC after two previous low transverse incisions, provided that the informed consent process presents the uncertainties of the evidence.
- Cephalocentesis is an ethically permissible form of intrapartum management for fetal hydrocephalus with severe associated anomalies.
- Non-aggressive obstetric management is ethically permissible when there is (1) a very high probability, but sometimes less than complete certainty, about the diagnosis and, (2) either very high probability of death or survival with a very high probability of severe and irreversible deficit of cognitive developmental capacity as a result of the anomaly diagnosed.

5 Planned home birth

5.1 Introduction

Planned home birth is now an established clinical practice in many countries. In the United States, this practice has increased by 29 %, from 2004 to 2009.[1,2] The American College of Obstetricians and Gynecologists (ACOG) has stated that pregnant women have a right to elect planned home birth.[3] The Royal College of Obstetricians and Gynaecologists (RCOG) goes further and explicitly endorses planned home birth.[4] These statements make the implicit assumption that planned home birth is compatible with professional responsibility for pregnant and fetal patients in the intrapartum period (occurring during childbirth). In this chapter we show that, from the perspective of the professional responsibility model of perinatal ethics, such an assumption lacks scientific and ethical justification and that, therefore, attendance at planned home birth is a violation of professional responsibility.[1,5]

Professional responsibility is an essential component of clinical ethics, including clinical ethics in planned home birth. On the basis of the professional responsibility model of perinatal ethics, we provide a critical appraisal of the assumption in the ACOG and RCOG statements that planned home birth is compatible with professional responsibility in obstetric care. We also show that the ineliminable, clinically unnecessary, and therefore clinically unacceptable intrinsic perinatal risks of the home setting mean that attendants at planned home birth, regardless of their training, cannot justifiably consider themselves to be professionals or claim to be engaging in professional obstetric care. We conclude by identifying the implications of the professional responsibility model for the response of perinatologists to expressions of interest in planned hospital birth by pregnant women.

5.2 Critical appraisal of the assumption that planned home birth is compatible with professional responsibility

As explained in Chapter 1, the professional responsibility model of perinatal ethics applies the ethical concept of medicine as a profession to obstetric care. The focus of this chapter is on planned home birth, which, by definition, occurs at the end of pregnancy. As also explained in Chapters 1 and 4, in the professional responsibility model, during the intrapartum period the perinatologist has two patients, the pregnant patient and the fetal patient, when the pregnant women presents for care. The perinatologist, therefore, has beneficence-based obligations to both the pregnant patient and fetal patient to protect and promote their health-related interests. The perinatologist also has autonomy-based obligations to the pregnant woman. These obligations focus on empowering the pregnant woman with information that she needs to make decisions with her obstetric healthcare professional about the responsible clinical management of her pregnancy. The perinatologist must in all cases take into account and balance beneficence-based and autonomy-based obligations to the pregnant patient and beneficence-based obligations to the fetal patient. This ethically complex relationship means that the fetal patient is not a separate patient, i.e. beneficence-based obligations to the fetal patient are a part of, but not the entirety of, the ethical relationship between the obstetric healthcare professional and the pregnant patient and fetal patient.[6]

ACOG sanctions the right of a pregnant woman to select the birth setting,[3] while RCOG goes further and explicitly endorses planned home birth.[4] Both statements implicitly assume that planned home birth is compatible with professional responsibility to the pregnant patient and fetal patient in the intrapartum period of term pregnancies. We disagree and turn now to a critical appraisal of this implicit assumption.

We do so on the basis of our analyses of planned home and new data analyses that were not available to either ACOG or RCOG. In previous analyses, we have shown that planned home birth, because the ineliminable risk of emergency transport of laboring women to the hospital, there is an increased risk of adverse perinatal outcomes.[7] We have also reported the results of a new analysis of the Centers for Disease Control's National Center for Health Statistics birth certificate data files for the period 2007–2010, that strongly corroborates our earlier analyses.[8] The resulting study population of more than 13 million births is the largest study population to date.

Our analysis focused on relative risk, the ratio of the probability of an event in the group exposed to a form of clinical management, planned home birth in this case, versus the probability of an event in the non-exposed group, hospital birth in this case. Relative-risk analysis is appropriate when the outcome measured has a low probability of occurrence. We demonstrated a relative risk of 10.55 for 5-minute Apgar scores of zero for home versus hospital birth, which increases to 14.24 for nulliparous women. The relative risk of seizures and other neurologic disorders was 3.80 for home versus hospital birth, which increased to 6.28 for nulliparous women.[8] Subsequently, we showed an increased risk of neonatal mortality from planned home birth. The absolute risk of total term neonatal mortality was 1.26/1,000 births with a relative risk of 3.87 when compared to midwife deliveries in the hospital. The relative risk increased to 6.74 for primaparous women and to 7.76 for women beyond 41 weeks.[9]

These increased risks result in clinically significant perinatal and neonatal mortality and morbidity, which can be prevented by hospital birth. These perinatal risks, therefore, become clinically unnecessary to impose on the fetal and neonatal patients, who cannot consent to them. There is an obvious beneficence-based obligation, and therefore professional responsibility to prevent such unnecessary clinical risks to fetal and neonatal patients when there is a safe and effective alternative. That alternative is a planned hospital birth, which, our analysis shows, significantly decreases perinatal morbidity and mortality. Given the clinically unnecessary violation of beneficence-based obligations to the fetal and neonatal patient, any claim that the home birth setting is compatible with professional integrity founders on these data.

In light of these data analysis and their ethical implications, it becomes apparent that the ACOG statement suffers from internal inconsistency. First, ACOG's position, in effect, holds that the pregnant woman's right to select her preferred birth setting at home should be recognized, even though ACOG recommends against planned home birth.[3] The ethical implication of the data analyses that we have just described is that one cannot sanction the right of a pregnant woman to select a birth setting that is inconsistent with professional integrity and responsibility without taking the view that such a right is unconstrained by professional integrity and responsibility. Yet ACOG is committed to the professional integrity of obstetric practice. Second, in sanctioning such a right, ACOG has implicitly invoked the maternal-rights-based reductionist model. In simultaneously recommending against planned home birth, ACOG has implicitly invoked the professional responsibility model. As is clear from the account of the two models in Chapter 1, the two models cannot be invoked simultaneously.

In light of these data analyses and their ethical implications, RCOG's problem is more serious. By endorsing planned home birth, RCOG has implicitly embraced the view that planned home birth is consistent with professional integrity and responsibility.[4] The clinically significant and unnecessary increased relative perinatal risks of planned home birth rule out such consistency.

As professional associations of obstetricians, ACOG and RCOG should be committed to the professional responsibility model of obstetric ethics. Our clinical and ethical analysis of the CDC data support the conclusion that planned home birth is not compatible with professional integrity, and therefore professional responsibility in patient care. In light of the new data analysis and its ethical implications, both ACOG and RCOG should reconsider their statements on planned home birth. RCOG now needs to justify its endorsement of planned birth both scientifically and ethically. Both ACOG and RCOG should unequivocally recommend against planned home birth. They should also be clear that no obstetrician should participate in planned home birth, because this would be facilitating clinically unnecessary, unsafe delivery, which is incompatible with professional integrity. Both ACOG and RCOG should be explicit that intentionally facilitating unsafe clinical practice of any kind is not permitted in professional medical practice.

ACOG now needs especially to justify scientifically and ethically its sanction of planned home birth, because, as planned home birth has increased in frequency, clinically unnecessary risks of adverse perinatal outcomes have also increased. Neither ACOG nor RCOG sanction a woman's right to smoke or consume spirit beverages during pregnancy and both explicitly recommend against these behaviors during pregnancy.[10,11] Any perinatologist who were to endorse or even sanction such clinically unsafe and unnecessary practices as smoking or drinking alcohol by pregnant patients would be justifiably regarded as acting inconsistently with professional responsibility. *Mutatis mutandis*, attendants at planned home birth, no matter their training or experience, should *not* be regarded as acting consistently with professional responsibility. It follows that planned home birth should not be endorsed or even sanctioned by any professional obstetric organization.

5.3 Planned home birth attendants are not acting in a professional capacity

The professional responsibility model of perinatal ethics has an important and heretofore unidentified implication for planned home birth. In light of these data analyses, planned home birth is not consistent with the first commitment in the ethical concept of medicine as a profession, the commitment to become and remain scientifically and clinically competent in patient care. (See Chapter 1) Scientifically and clinically competent provision of perinatal care requires the capacity to diagnose and prevent obstetric complications. Scientifically and clinically competent provision of perinatal care also requires the ability to diagnose and respond quickly and effectively to unexpected obstetric emergencies. No such capacities exist in planned home birth. This clinical reality is not a function of who the attendant is. Instead, the setting of planned home birth is itself determinative, because, given limited diagnostic and treatment capacity and especially the high and highly variable transport times, there is no assured access to the hospital-based advances in obstetric practices that have greatly improved maternal, fetal, and neonatal outcomes of unexpected obstetric complications and emergencies over the past century. The implication is clear and, unfortunately, stark: Any claim by an attendant to planned home birth to be providing scientifically and clinically competent obstetric services is altogether implausible.[1,5]

The second commitment of the ethical concept of medicine as a profession requires healthcare professionals to protect and promote the health-related interests of patients as the primary concern and motivation, keeping self-interest systematically secondary. The inability to provide scientifically and clinical competent perinatal care in the home setting of planned home birth means that it is not possible for this commitment to be met. This conclusion also has a clear and, unfortunately, stark implication for attendants at planned home birth: they cannot plausibly claim to be acting primarily in the health-related interests of pregnant women, fetuses, and neonates.

These two implications of the new data analysis are, we freely admit, jarring. Together, these two implications support a third clear and, unfortunately stark, implication: no one who attends a planned home birth can with scientific, clinical, and ethical justification claim the title of being a "professional." This applies equally to physicians, certified nurse midwives, and those who represent themselves as professional or licensed midwives. Because it is not justified to describe attendants at home birth as professionals, no matter their training or experience, neither the pregnant woman nor the neonate can justifiably be referred to as "patients." The pregnant woman becomes merely a client in a contractual, not professional, relationship. This is the nature of the non-professional relationship that results from the rights-based reductionist model of obstetric ethics. There are associations of professional midwives and they have codes of ethics.[12,13] Having such a code is usually one of the defining features of a profession. This is not the case for code of ethics of associations of attendants at planned home birth. These codes of ethics cannot plausibly be represented to pregnant women or to the public as *professional* codes of ethics.

5.4 Professional responsibility and hospital birth

The professional responsibility model of perinatal ethics has important implications for clinical practice. First and foremost, when a pregnant woman is transported to the hospital from a planned home birth, she should receive uniformly excellent perinatal care. The second component of the ethical concept of medicine as a profession requires the entire obstetric team to focus on the patient and not themselves. This means that judgmental attitudes should not be cultivated and that judgmental statements should never be made. Because they would be self-indulging, such attitudes and statements would be patently inconsistent with professional responsibility.

The professional responsibility model of perinatal ethics also calls for continuous enhancement of the organizational culture of hospital-based obstetric care. First and foremost, the professional responsibility model calls for an organizational culture of safety and preventing clinically unnecessary intervention.[14] Patient safety has become the paramount goal of hospital-based obstetrics over the past decade. This change has required reforming organizational culture and includes the adoption of team principles and safety drills.[14] Adopting a comprehensive safety culture has been shown to reduce the rate of cesarean delivery.[15] Adopting a comprehensive safety culture has become an important means for responding effectively to the concerns of pregnant women about excessive obstetric interventions in the hospital setting. These improvements implement the first commitment of the ethical concept of medicine as a profession. The majority of these safety goals cannot be satisfactorily implemented at a planned home birth. While the team concept in the hospital includes multidisciplinary members, such as certified nurse midwives, nurses, anesthesiologists, pediatricians, obstetricians, there is no team concept at a planned home birth. At a planned home birth, there is almost always only one attendant assisting the pregnant woman with her delivery. As a consequence, team training cannot occur, much less become a component of planned home birth, which is not compatible with quality obstetric care. None of the clinical benefits of well-trained team case accrue to pregnant women, fetuses, and newborns in the planned home birth setting.[16] Indeed, the increased relative risk of clinically preventable, and therefore unnecessary outcomes that we have documented underscores this point.

The second commitment of the ethical concept of medicine as a profession requires the creation of an organizational culture of compassion that supports the preferences of pregnant women throughout their pregnancies and aims to maximize a home-like setting in the hospital. For example, there should be self-conscious, deliberate efforts to create a quiet setting on labor and delivery and postpartum floors.[14]

5.5 Respect for the pregnant women's rights

There are two ways in which respect for women's rights should be understood. The first starts with the right of the woman to make decisions and control what happens to her body. The physician is bound to acknowledge and implement the patient's preferences, without constraint. This is a purely contractual model of the physician-patient relationship in which the woman protects herself by the exercise of her autonomy-based rights. "In a democratic society, a woman has the right to choose where she might undergo one of the most important experiences of her life, and where she will begin to bond with a child she will raise lovingly."[17]

As described in Chapter 1, this is maternal rights-based reductionism, in which the patient's rights systematically override professional responsibility. In the resulting contractual relationship, the physician's obligation to protect the pregnant woman, much less the fetal and neonatal patient, is completely subordinated to the pregnant woman's rights. In the professional relationship called for by the professional responsibility model of perinatal ethics, the perinatologist has an independent ethical obligation, as a matter of professional integrity, to protect pregnant, fetal, and neonatal patients. As explained in Chapter 1, these beneficence-based obligations must, in all cases, be balanced against autonomy-based obligations to the pregnant patient. Beneficence-based and autonomy-based obligations combine to create the professional responsibility to empower the pregnant woman to make informed decisions about the management of her pregnancy and care of her newborn child. The physician's role is to identify and present medically reasonable alternatives for the management of pregnancy, i.e. clinical management for which there is an evidence base of net clinical benefit. In a professional relationship, the physician's integrity justifiably limits the woman's rights by limiting the scope of clinically reasonable alternatives. This limitation does not exist in the rights-based reductionist model of women's rights.

In the professional responsibility model of perinatal ethics, the pregnant woman has the right to select from among the medically reasonable alternatives.

If she rejects them all and also remains a patient, then her refusal is not a simple exercise of a negative right to non-interference. Her refusal is more complex, because it is coupled with a positive right to the services of clinicians and the resources of healthcare organizations and society.[18] In all ethical theories, positive rights come with limits. In the clinical setting, ethically justified limits originate in professional integrity, because professional integrity prohibits provision of clinical management that is not safe.

In summary, from the perspective of the professional responsibility model of perinatal ethics, insistence on implementing the unconstrained rights of the pregnant woman to control the birth location is an ethical error and therefore has no place in professional perinatal practice. An editorial in *Lancet* succinctly summarized this point: "Women have the right to choose how and where to give birth, but they do not have the right to put their baby at risk."[19]

5.6 Professionally appropriate responses

5.6.1 What should perinatologists do to address the root cause of the recrudescence of planned home birth?

The first professional responsibility of perinatologists is to ensure that hospital delivery is safe, respectful, and compassionate.[14,20,21] Current, inappropriate practices may be fueling the recrudescence of planned home birth. Physician leaders need to closely scrutinize organizational policies and practices and should see to it that staffing is competent and adequate. Well-trained, compassionate in-house attending obstetrical and anesthesia coverage should be required for all hospitals offering planned hospital delivery. Unnecessary obstetric interventions need to be assiduously prevented by adherence to evidence-based guidelines. Teaching of noninvasive care and mode of delivery should become an essential part of training. Physician leaders must be especially watchful for trends of clinically unjustified increased intervention that results from inappropriate self-interest in reducing liability, convenience, or financial gain.[22,23] This focus on maternal and fetal safety should be complemented with an emphasis on compassionate care that respects the pregnant woman as a person by acknowledging and striving to meet her psychosocial needs. Birth centers with immediate access to cesarean delivery, as well as collaborative practice models between perinatologists and nurse midwives should be encouraged.[24–29] The goal should be effective integration of clinically competent and compassionate obstetric care as presaged by the Scottish physician-ethicist John Gregory, more than two centuries ago, who called for physicians to be scientifically excellent and to exhibit "gentleness of manners, and a compassionate heart," what Shakespeare calls "the milk of human kindness."[30]

5.6.2 How should perinatologists respond when a woman raises the topic of planned home birth?

The increased risks of planned home birth described above are preventable by planned hospital delivery. Planned home birth should not be considered medically reasonable in deliberative clinical judgment. This clinical judgment should be respectfully communicated and the woman's questions addressed in an evidence-based fashion. The pregnant woman should be informed of the high transport rate and the increased, preventable risks to herself, her fetus, and her baby, as well as the psychosocial harms of emergency transport. The perinatologist should recommend strongly against planned home birth and obtain informed consent for delivery in a safe and compassionate hospital environment or a birth center with immediate hospital access.

5.6.3 How should perinatologists respond to a woman's request for the perinatologist to participate in planned home birth?

For a woman who is nonetheless committed to planned home birth, the perinatologist should explain that professional responsibility prohibits participation in or facilitation of substandard clinical care. As explained in Chapter 1, the simple fact that a pregnant patient has made a request does not by itself create a professional responsibility to implement that request, especially when the request is for clinical management that is not medically reasonable.

5.6.4 How should perinatologists respond when a patient is received on emergency transport from a planned home birth?

There is a strict professional obligation to provide excellent medical care in *all* obstetric emergencies, no matter how they originated. Without hesitation, therefore, the perinatologist should provide excellent, compassionate, emergency obstetric care to all pregnant women transported from planned home birth. Perinatologists have a compassion-based obligation to be aware of and address the psychosocial harms of such transport, in an attempt to ameliorate their long-term effects.

5.6.5 Should obstetricians participate in or refer patients to a randomized controlled clinical trial of planned home vs. planned hospital birth?

The analysis above of the safety data on home birth shows that there is an unacceptable increased risk of perinatal morbidity and morality and neonatal morality.

Equipoise, an important ethical condition for initiating randomized controlled trials, implies genuine uncertainty as to whether one treatment is better than another. For home birth, equipoise does not exist, because a controlled clinical trial with home birth as one arm would subject pregnant, fetal, and neonatal patients to preventable, unnecessary risk of mortality, morbidity, and disability when compared to hospital delivery. The fundamental ethical imperative in research with human subjects is to protect them from impermissible harm.[31] This imperative would be violated by a randomized controlled clinical trial. This conclusion is made all the stronger when one realizes that fetal and neonatal patients are vulnerable subjects of research because they are incapable of consent, and therefore cannot protect themselves. Randomized controlled clinical trials of planned home vs. planned hospital birth violate research ethics. It is, therefore, impermissible for an obstetrician to participate in or refer patients to such trials.

5.7 Conclusion

Advocacy of planned home birth is a compelling example of what happens when ideology replaces professionally disciplined clinical judgment and policy. Perinatologists should eschew maternal rights-based reductionism in the professional ethics of planned home birth and replace maternal rights-based reductionism with the professional responsibility model of perinatal ethics.

5.8 References

1. Chervenak FA, McCullough LB, Brent RL, Levene LI, Arabin B. Planned home birth: the professional responsibility response. Am J Obstet Gynecol 2013;208:31–38.
2. MacDorman MF, Matthews TJ, Lequerq E. Home births in the united states: 1990–2009, NCHS Data Brief 84. January 2012:1–8.
3. American College of Obstetricians and Gynecologists. Committee Opinion No. 476. Committee on Obstetric Practice. Planned home birth. Obstet Gynecol 2011;117:425–428.
4. Royal College of Obstetricians and Gynaecologists and Royal College of Midwives Joint Statement No. 2. April, 2007. Home births, available at www.rcog.org.uk/files/rcog-corp/uploaded-files/JointStatmentHomeBirths2007.pdf, accessed March 8, 2014.
5. Chervenak FA, McCullough LB, Grünebaum A Arabin B, Levene MI, Brent RL. Planned home birth in the United States and professionalism: a critical assessment. J Clin Ethics 2013;24:184–191.
6. McCullough LB, Chervenak FA. Ethics in Obstetrics and Gynecology. New York: Oxford University Press, 1994.
7. Chervenak FA, McCullough LB. Obstetric ethics: an essential dimension of planned home birth. Obstet Gynecol 2011;117:1183–1187.
8. Grünebaum A, McCullough LB, Sapra KJ, Brent RL, Levene MI, Arabin B, Chervenak FA. Apgar score of zero at five minutes and seizures or serious neonatal dysfunction in relation to birth setting. Am J Obstet Gynecol 2013;209:323.e1–6.

9. Grünebaum A, McCullough LB, Sapra KJ, Brent RL, Levene MI, Arabin B, Chervenak FA. Early and total neonatal mortality in relation to birth setting in the United States, 2006–2009. Am J Obstet Gynecol: in press.
10. American College of Obstetricians and Gynecologists. Committee Opinion No. 316. Committee on Health Care for Underserved Women; ACOG Committee on Obstetric Practice. Smoking cessation during pregnancy. Obstet Gynecol 2005;104:883–888.
11. Royal College of Obstetricians and Gynaecologists, RCOG Statement on paper 'Maternal smoking during pregnancy and criminal offending among adult offspring'. November 16, 2010. Available at www.rcog.org.uk/what-we-do/campaigning-and-opinions/statement/rcog-statement-paper-%E2 %80 %98maternal-smoking-during-pregnanc, accessed February 26, 2014.
12. American College of Nurse Midwives. Code of Ethics. Available at www.midwife.org/siteFiles/descriptive/code_of_ethics_2008.pdf, accessed March 8, 2014.
13. The Association of Texas Midwives. Code of Ethical Midwifery Practice. Available at www.texasmidwives.com/PDFfiles/ATM%20Code%20of%20Ethics_Original.pdf, accessed March 8, 2014.
14. Grünebaum A, Chervenak F, Skupski D. Effect of a comprehensive patient safety program on compensation payments and sentinel events. Am J Obstet Gynecol 2011;204:97–105.
15. Grünebaum A, Dudenhausen J, Chervenak FA, Skupski D. Reduction of cesarean delivery rates after implementation of a comprehensive patient safety program. J Perinatal Med 2013;41:51–55.
16. Chervenak FA, McCullough LB, Grünebaum A Arabin B, Levene MI, Brent RL. Planned home birth: a violation of the best interests of the child standard? Pediatrics 2013;132:921–923.
17. Zohar N, quoted in Even D. Health ministry delaying delivery of new restrictions on at-home births. Haaretz January 3, 2012, available at www.haaretz.com/print-edition/news/health-ministry-delaying-delivery-of-new-restrictions-on-at-home-births-1.405164, accessed March 8, 2014.
18. Chervenak FA, McCullough LB. Justified limits on refusal of intervention. Hastings Cent Rep 1991;21:12–18.
19. Home birth – proceed with caution. Lancet 2010:376:303.
20. Knox GE, Simpson KR. Perinatal high reliability. Am J Obstet Gynecol 2011;204:373–377.
21. Pettker CM, Thung SF, Raab CA, Donahue KP, Copel JA, Lockwood CJ, Funai EF. A comprehensive obstetrics patient safety program improves safety climate and culture. Am J Obstet Gynecol 2011;204:216.e1–6.
22. Chervenak FA, McCullough LB. The moral foundation of medical leadership: the professional virtues of the physician as fiduciary of the patient. Am J Obstet Gynecol 2001;184:875–880.
23. Chervenak FA, McCullough LB, Brent RL. The professional responsibility model of physician leadership. Am J Obstet Gynecol 2013;208:97–101.
24. Hodnett ED, Downe S, Edwards N, Walsh D. Home-like versus conventional institutional settings for birth. Cochrane Database Syst Rev 2005;(1).
25. Hodnett ED, Gates S, Hofmeyr GJ, Sakala C. Continuous support for women during childbirth. Cochrane Database Syst Rev 2007;(3).
26. Shaw-Battista J, Fineberg A, Boehler B, et al. Obstetrician and nurse-midwife collaboration. Obstet Gynecol 2011;118:6630672.
27. Darlington A, McBroom K, Warnick S. A Northwest collaborative practice model. Obstet Gynecol 2011;118:673–677.
28. Hutchison MS, Ennis L, Shaw-Battista J, et al. Great minds don't think alike: collaborative maternity care at San Francisco General Hospital. Obstet Gynecol 2011;118:678–682.
29. DeJoy S, Burkman RT, Graves BW, et al. Making it work: successful collaborative practice. Obstet Gynecol 2011;118:683–686.
30. Gregory J. Lectures on the Duties and Qualifications of a Physician. London: W. Strahan and T. Cadell, 1772. Reprinted in McCullough LB, ed. John Gregory's Writings on Medical Ethics

and Philosophy of Medicine. Dordrecht, Netherlands: Kluwer Academic Publishers 1998:161–245.
31. Brody BA, McCullough LB, Sharp RR. Consensus and controversy in clinical research ethics. JAMA 2005;294:1411–1414.

5.9 Summary Points

- In response to expressions of interest in planned home birth by pregnant women, the perinatologist should explain its perinatal and neonatal risks, recommend strongly against planned home birth, and recommend hospital birth strongly.
- Perinatologists should not participate in planned home birth because doing so is incompatible with the professional responsibility model of perinatal ethics.
- The perinatologist should be non-judgmental and provide excellent medical care to women and babies transferred to the hospital after maternal, fetal, or neonatal complications of planned home birth.
- The professional responsibility model of perinatal ethics requires obstetricians to address and remedy legitimate dissatisfaction of pregnant women with some hospital settings. Creating a sustained culture of comprehensive safety, which cannot be achieved in planned home birth, informed by compassionate and respectful treatment of pregnant women, should be a primary focus of professional perinatal responsibility.
- Perinatologists should not participate in or refer patients to randomized controlled trials of planned home birth vs. hospital birth, because the requirement of equipoise is not met.

6 Pregnant patients with mental disorders

6.1 Introduction

The care of pregnant patients with mental disorders poses particularly difficult clinical ethical challenges to the perinatologist. These challenges center mainly on the patient's capacity for decision making which can be adversely affected by depression or psychosis even when it is well controlled by medication. Perinatologists, for good reason, become uncertain what weight to give to patients' preferences when decision-making capacity is impaired, e.g. by flat affect, lack of insight, auditory hallucinations, delusional thinking, impaired thought processes, or even by the very denial of pregnancy itself. These ethical challenges become more pronounced when the perinatologist is concerned that the patient is making decisions that do not take adequate account of such factors as the effect of her mental disorder on her decision-making capacity, her ability to cooperate with a plan for obstetric care, her vulnerability to control by others, and the limits of sometimes fragile social circumstances.

This chapter provides a clinically based, ethical framework for managing the challenges of decision making with this population of pregnant patients. We then deploy this framework to guide judicious decision making by patients and perinatalogists regarding the continuation or termination of previable pregnancies and regarding intrapartum care, especially cesarean delivery.[1]

6.2 Clinical considerations

Schizophrenia, which has a lifetime risk of around 0.5 to 1 percent, is a chronic mental disorder that has a median age of onset in the late twenties for women.[2,3] Women with schizophrenia have the same average number of pregnancies as non-mentally ill controls.[4] To the best of our knowledge, the prevalence of schizophrenia among pregnant women has not been determined, but, given the age of onset, obstetricians will see these patients in their practices.

The mode of onset of schizophrenia and course of illness, including symptoms, can vary markedly among patients. However, active-phase symptoms commonly include bizarre delusions, hallucinations, and disorganized thinking, speech, and behavior. Recurrence of acute-phase symptoms is common whereas complete remission is not.[2] Depression, or elevation in mood associated with irritability, may also complicate the course.

Female patients with schizophrenia constitute a particularly vulnerable population. Many patients live in homeless or impoverished circumstances, have unrecognized physical illnesses[5,6] and experience difficulties in establishing and maintaining stable relationships, including those with a male partner. Sexually active female patients with major mental disorders including schizophrenia are more likely than controls to report having had more than one sexual partner over the preceding year[4,7] and to report having been coerced into unwanted sexual activity.[7,8] These patients also sustain a greater risk than controls for sexually transmitted diseases, including HIV infection and AIDS, and for both unplanned and unwanted pregnancies.[4,7]

Rates of obstetric complications,[9,10] congenital malformations and perinatal deaths[11,12] are also higher, although not substantially so, in women with schizophrenia than the general population. Women with schizophrenia are particularly vulnerable to physical abuse during pregnancy.[3] Furthermore, there is evidence that patients with major mental disorders, including schizophrenia, are more likely to have induced abortions than non-psychotic women.[4,7] Many patients who carry their pregnancies through to term eventually lose custody of their children, either to family members or to child protective services that arrange for foster care or adoption.[7,13] Repeat pregnancies for this population of patients are common.[7] Alcohol and illicit drug use, which is more prevalent in psychiatric patient populations,[14] may contribute to the risks for unwanted pregnancies, sexually transmitted infections, and to obstetric complications. Impaired decision making capacity is another factor that might contribute to the risk of unwanted pregnancies, sexually transmitted diseases, or to being sexually or physically abused.

In the past, many of these patients were committed to long-term psychiatric institutions. The process of deinstitutionalization of the mentally ill over the past four decades has resulted in patients with schizophrenia no longer being segregated from the rest of society. This process has also been associated with markedly increased opportunities for sexual encounters and increased fertility rates among women with schizophrenia.[15] The associated risks of pregnancy, including the management of complications and decisions about termination of pregnancy, have therefore increasingly become matters of concern to obstetricians.

As a result of deinstitutionalization, women with schizophrenia are usually cared for by psychiatrists and other mental health professionals in outpatient settings. These professionals will refer patients who become pregnant to obstetricians for the management of pregnancy, including termination of pregnancy. Sometimes, however, mental health professionals fail to address contraceptive issues or to take adequate sexual histories, which can lead to delayed recognition of pregnancy.[16,17] Failure to recognize pregnancy on the part of a mental health professional, or to accept pregnancy by a patient, can lead to referral at later stages or even near or during the intrapartum period. In particular, precipitous delivery and, in rare cases, infanticide have been associated with psychotic denial of pregnancy.[18]

6.3 Responsibly managing the decision-making process

The proposed ethical framework comprises five elements: an account of the concept of chronically and variably impaired autonomy and its implications for schizophrenia; assisted decision making to enhance the ability of patients to identify and assess consequences of their decisions, based on their own values and beliefs; surrogate decision making; strategies for dealing with the strong feelings that these patients can evoke and any subsequent tendency to make decisions for, rather than with, these patients; and the concept of the fetus as a patient, which is described in Chapter 1. The focus of this framework is on preventive ethics, i.e. devising clinical strategies that anticipate and seek to prevent ethical conflict in the decision-making process about the management of pregnancy.[19]

6.3.1 Chronically and variably impaired autonomy

Patients exercise their capacity for autonomous decision making in a stepwise process.[20,21] We emphasize that impairments in any one step will adversely affect the patient's ability to complete subsequent steps. The seven steps are as follows:

1. The patient attends to the information that is provided to her by the physician.
2. The patient absorbs, retains, and recalls this information as needed in the subsequent steps.
3. The patient can reason from present events to their future likely consequences, which is called cognitive understanding.[22]
4. The patient understands that these consequences could happen to her and/or her fetus and future child, should her pregnancy continue to delivery. This is called appreciation.[23]
5. The patient assesses these consequences on the basis of her own values and beliefs, which is called evaluative understanding.[22]
6. The patient expresses a voluntary decision for or against offered or recommended clinical management. "Voluntary" means that the decision is not subject to substantial control by external factors (other people) or internal factors (such as auditory hallucinations).[24]
7. The patient can, when requested, explain her decision on the basis of her cognitive and evaluative understanding.

Psychosis during pregnancy can impair Steps 1 and 2, when attention and absorption, recall, or retention of information are adversely affected by auditory hallucinations or paranoia, both of which can significantly distract the patient. Depression may prevent the patient from turning her attention to what the perinatologist is telling her. Cognitive understanding and appreciation can be adversely affected by lack of insight or by psychotic denial of pregnancy. Evaluative understanding can be adversely affected by discounting the positive aspects of one's future or by paranoia. This might include paranoid beliefs about medication (e.g. that it is poison), about health care professionals (e.g. that they intend to harm, not help, the patient), and about the fetus (e.g. that the fetus is emanating "bad vibrations" or that the fetus is somehow alien and needs to be expelled from her body). The patient's ability to make a voluntary decision (Step 6) can be impaired by hearing voices that may, for example, command a patient, alternatively, to hurt herself, hurt the fetus, terminate the pregnancy, or continue the pregnancy. Steps 6 and 7 can also be adversely affected by formal thought disorders, including looseness of associations that can sometimes be quite marked, or severe ambivalence and lack of stable preferences.

These adverse effects of mental disorders on the seven steps of decision making may display marked variation across patients and, over time, within a single patient. This variability, which can include normal function, is one of the defining features of mental disorders, as we have emphasized above. This variation also appears in the wide range of responses of patients to medication. Moreover, mental disorders are chronic conditions, sometimes punctuated by acute decompensation.

In the language of ethics, mental disorders can result in chronically and variably impaired autonomy.[20,21] Mental disorders can, over time, disrupt one or more of the seven steps of exercising the capacity for autonomous decision making and to varying degrees. This is in contrast to severe and profound cognitive disability, where the loss of autonomy is nearly complete and displays little variation. Depending on the severity of their mental illness and the clinical intervention and support of their psychiatrist and perinatologist, many, if not most, of these pregnant patients can exercise their capacity for autonomous decision making to an adequate degree.

6.3.2 Assisted decision making

The first response to diminished decision-making capacity resulting from chronically and variably impaired autonomy should be to reverse such diminishments so that the patient can make her own decisions. The primary justification of assisted decision making is to prevent unwarranted paternalistic intrusion onto the decision-making by physicians, family members, institutions, and the state. Another justification is to avoid flying a false flag of autonomy, i.e. taking uncritically the preferences of patients with significant impairments, especially their refusal to cooperate with a proposed plan of care.

While first-trimester exposure to low potency antipsychotic medications may lead to a small increase in the risk of congenital malformations, less is known about higher potency and newer antipsychotic agents.[25] Nevertheless, medications used to treat mental disorders, when safe for the fetus, can be used as the initial response to impaired decision-making capacity. The time window within which these medications become beneficial varies. Impairments in the early steps of the decision making process, especially those caused by hallucinations, are responsive to medication. The systemic effects of early-step impairments of attention and absorption, retention and recall and later-step impairments of appreciation can thereby be alleviated or even eliminated with subsequent systematic improvement of decision-making capacity. Pharmacologic intervention can also enhance the capacity for voluntary decision making by reducing or eliminating such factors as diminished sense of self-worth and self-efficacy, hallucinatory commands, or unreasoning fear of the fetus.

Psychosocial interventions, such as communication-skills training and problem-solving strategies, combined with optimal pharmacologic management should also be considered.[26] These strategies should be targeted toward proactive consideration of decisions about the management of pregnancy and possible complications, to enhance cognitive understanding, and to help the patient to achieve more stable values and beliefs about her health care generally, and the management of her pregnancy. Enhancing the patient's communication skills also helps her to become a more effective advocate for her own preferences, thus reducing the possibility of coercion by family members or health care professionals.

The perinatologist should undertake education of the pregnant woman about the clinical issues at stake, including the option of termination of pregnancy and, for pregnancies going to term, subsequent clinical management and the nature of her psychiatric diagnosis and its related impairments of decision-making capacity. Obviously, such education can enhance cognitive understanding; and more complete cognitive understanding helps to improve evaluative understanding. Increased cognitive understanding of one's own mental illness can lead to improved insight into how that mental illness affects one's life and decisions. That is, patients can be assisted by education to achieve increased insight into their own condition and decisions, thus enhancing their appreciation.

6.3.3 Surrogate decision making

Impairments of cognitive understanding mean that there will be impairments of evaluative understanding in that the patient's ability to assess consequences is a function of her awareness of those consequences and appreciation that those consequences could happen in her life. However, such impairments do not mean that patients with serious impairments have no values and cannot to any extent express preferences based on them. These values and preferences can be elicited from the patient. Information about the patient's premorbid values can be elicited from those who know the patient well, especially family members, as is done routinely for patients whose medical condition results in lost decision-making capacity. This information can then be taken into account in surrogate decision making that assesses the consequences for the patient based on her values. This is an important alternative to the unacceptably paternalistic approach of decisions by others about what values should be imposed on the patient.[19]

To elicit patients' values, it is useful to ask them what is important to them.[27] Patients with mental illness can sometimes answer this question in a way that reports relatively stable and enduring values, even if they are significantly impaired in other aspects of decision making. These values should then be used by the surrogate decision maker, along with information from others about the patient's values, to make decisions for the patient. This approach puts into practice the substituted judgment standard of surrogate decision making, according to which the surrogate should, to the extent possible, make the decision that the patient would make, were the patient able to do so.[28]

Some patients will not be able to answer questions about what is important to them consistently. Patients with significantly reduced appreciation are especially vulnerable to this deficit. For example, a patient who thinks that the fetus is a predator will probably say that it is important to get rid of the predator. A patient in denial of her pregnancy, a phenomenon that waxes and wanes over time, will not be able to take account of the effects of her behavior on the health of the fetus at times when she is strongly denying the pregnancy.[18] For these patients, in the absence of reliable information from others about their values, surrogate decision making should be guided by the best interests standard.[28] This standard calls for the surrogate to make decisions that protect and promote the patient's health-related interests. In all cases, physicians should identify the legally appropriate surrogate decision maker, which can vary from jurisdiction to jurisdiction.

6.3.4 Strategies for dealing with strong feelings that these patients can evoke

Sometimes these patients can generate strong feelings on the part of physicians because they may lack stable preferences, a problem that can become compounded by irreversible chronically and variably impaired autonomy. Physicians may also have substantial concerns about the risks at stake for the pregnant woman, for her fetus, and for her prospective child. Lack of stable preferences can lead to frustration with the patient and, if not disciplined appropriately, can support an inclination to make decisions for, not with, these patients and their surrogates. Concerns about risk tend to focus on the woman's capacity to rear a child, e.g. when the patient exhibits lack of engagement with social contacts and other forms of support that are crucial to child-rearing or when the patient has many previous illness episodes that have necessitated hospitalization. These concerns can create a sense of frustration that the woman may make decisions that are not in line with the physician's well-founded clinical judgments about the woman's ability and willingness to respond consistently to a newborn's behavior cues, such as crying when hungry or uncomfortable. These concerns can also create a sense of foreboding that the future child's safety may be jeopardized and that, if this problem becomes serious, the woman will experience considerable psychosocial loss should the courts take custody of her child.

The problem with such strong feelings is that they can unhinge clinical judgment from evidence, by supporting the assumption that mental illness per se makes someone incapable of being an adequate parent. Many of these women can successfully parent their children, given adequate ongoing social support and psychiatric care. Even in cases in which women have lost custody of their children due to child neglect or abuse, evaluation of parenting competency of mentally ill individuals is rarely clear-cut, and some mothers may raise subsequent children successfully.[29] Socio-economic factors may be more reliable predictors of parenting capacity than a psychiatric diagnosis.

Perinatologists should arrange for thorough assessment of the future parenting capacity by adequately trained professionals, using accepted methods for doing so.[30,31] Deficits can thus be identified in advance and addressed through education and training. In addition, obstetricians should also work with colleagues in social work to qualify the woman for available public and private community support, to mitigate limiting socio-economic factors.

This is a patient population at increased risk of alcohol and substance abuse. Drug and excessive alcohol use during pregnancy can provoke perhaps the strongest feelings of all unhealthy behaviors of pregnant women. Drug and excessive alcohol use can be viewed partly as moral issues, i.e. matters of bad choices, and partly as medical matters, i.e. the consequences of exposing the human central nervous system to potentially addicting substances. Perinatologists should regard such risk, in all cases, as multifactorial, and therefore resist the inclination to reduce the risk to any single factor. The clinical advantage of this multifactorial approach is that it supports a comprehensive, directive response to drug and alcohol use during pregnancy. This response should begin with an exploration of the patient's motivations, education about the risks of substance abuse, and assistance in changing attitudes and behaviors that could harm herself or her fetus. The professional responsibility model of perinatal ethics calls for the perinatologist to recommend abstinence, or at least minimizing consumption, during the course of pregnancy. Such a directive approach enhances and does not diminish or disrespect patient autonomy. This comprehensive, directive clinical response is, in our judgment, a powerful antidote to the very strong feelings of frustration and real foreboding that the combination of mental illness and substance abuse generates.

The general strategy for responding to strong feelings that these patients can evoke is two-fold: increasing one's commitment to deliberative clinical judgment, which includes the corrective of basing clinical judgment on evidence, and initiating interventions to address chronically and variably impaired autonomy. The goal of this strategy is to support the woman's autonomy-based prerogative to make well-informed decisions for herself about a healthy pregnancy and responsible child rearing, including the decision whether to raise her child or place her child for adoption. In this way, she is prepared to make decisions for herself that command the respect of those responsible for her care, thus undercutting the paternalistic tendency to make decisions for her that the strong feelings described above can evoke.

6.4 Clinical applications

6.4.1 The decision whether to continue a previable pregnancy to viability and thus to term

The preceding ethical framework generates guiding ethical considerations for clinical judgment and counseling pregnant women with psychoses about termination of previable pregnancies. As explained in Chapter 1, the previable fetus is a patient as a function of the pregnant woman's autonomy. The pregnant woman should be assumed to possess decision-making capacity. The perinatologist should be aware of feelings he or she may have in response to the patient and prevent those feelings from interfering with or distorting clinical judgment.

The perinatologist should undertake a careful assessment of the patient's ability to participate in the steps of decision making described above, to determine whether and how the patient exhibits chronically and variably impaired autonomy. For impairments that are identified, the patient should be offered treatment in an attempt to reverse the impairment and return the patient to threshold decision-making capacity.

When this goal cannot be accomplished, surrogate decision making becomes necessary. The substituted judgment standard calls for such decisions to be based, as much as possible, on the patient's values and beliefs. The surrogate should be assisted, as needed, to distinguish between his or her own values and beliefs and those of the patient, especially concerning the independent moral status of the fetus.

When the patient's values and beliefs are not known well enough to implement the substituted judgment standard, the best interests standard should be followed.[28] With rare exceptions, termination of pregnancy cannot be justified on the grounds of protecting the woman's health. The risks to the fetus of continuing pregnancy may be serious but with unreliable predictability. Given the nature of fetal anomalies that occur in this patient population,[11,12] the best interests standard, applied to the fetus, cannot, as a rule, justify termination. A surrogate decision for termination of pregnancy on grounds of the woman's or the fetus's interests, therefore, should not be accepted by the physician as authoritative.

6.4.2 Intrapartum management

The preceding ethical framework generates guiding ethical considerations for clinical judgment and counseling of the pregnant woman during intrapartum management. During the intrapartum period, the fetus is a patient. The perinatologist and pregnant woman, when she is presented for care, therefore, both have beneficence-based obligations to protect fetal life and health when doing so involves reasonable risks for the pregnant woman. The pregnant woman should be presumed to possess decision-making capacity. The perinatologist should be aware of feelings he or she may have in response to the patient and prevent those feelings from interfering with or distorting clinical judgment.

Decision making during the intrapartum period occurs under time constraints that become increasingly stringent as labor progresses. These time constraints, however, should not become an excuse for not engaging the pregnant woman in decisions about intrapartum management – any more than they should for any pregnant woman.

Intrapartum decision making can be enhanced by adopting the preventive ethics strategy of talking to the pregnant woman in advance about the fact that pregnancy can become high risk quickly and without warning, and eliciting her general views about cesarean delivery for fetal or maternal indications. (See Chapter 4) The physician should be willing to negotiate general considerations that the woman would accept as justifying aggressive obstetric management, such as fetal monitoring or cesarean delivery. There should also be frank discussion with the patient about the fact that maternal or fetal indications may become so compelling that her refusal of intervention, should it reflect impaired decision making with no time to address that impairment, will be overridden. The goal is to be in a position, as the patient's physician, to implement agreements already made that would justify not accepting significantly impaired refusal of intervention for maternal or fetal indications. This approach is known as a "Ulysses contract" in which the patient agrees to clinical management and agrees to have her later refusal of it ignored.

Matters become more complicated in the case of intrapartum decision making when the woman's first prenatal visit occurs during the intrapartum period. Precipitous delivery with no prenatal care is high-risk by definition. It is also more likely that the pregnant woman's depression has not been well managed and that the impairments of chronically and variably autonomy from psychosis may be more severe. When cesarean delivery is indicated for fetal benefit, including when the woman is unable to cooperate with labor and vaginal delivery, the physician should attempt to gain the patient's agreement to anesthesia, followed by cesarean delivery. If she refuses but is not physically resistant, anesthesia should be administered and cesarean delivery performed on the grounds that her obligation to take reasonable risks for fetal benefit takes precedence over "respect" for significantly impaired autonomy.[19,32]

6.4.3 Decisions about child-rearing and adoption

The ability to rear a child oneself is distinct from the ability to make decisions about the management of pregnancy; the latter are, arguably, medically more complex than the former. In addition, physicians possess no special expertise to evaluate a woman's ability to adequately rear a child. In addition, her chances of success are also a function of her support network and other social factors. The presumption should be that she is capable, with appropriate support, of childrearing. The burden of proof rests with clinical judgment that she lacks such capacity. The physician's concerns about lack of child-rearing capacity should be conveyed to social work colleagues, who have expertise in this area. If their evaluation supports these concerns, legal review should be sought under applicable law. Democratic societies have vested in judges the legal authority to determine who is fit to rear a child in ways consistent with protecting and promoting the child's interests.

6.5 Conclusion

Pregnant patients with mental disorders constitute a particularly vulnerable and clinically challenging population with regard to impairments of decision-making capacity, being controlled by others, unaddressed medical problems, and fragile social circumstances. We have proposed preventive ethics strategies, including assisted and surrogate decision making, and dealing with strong feelings that these patients can evoke. These strategies are designed to enhance and implement the patient's autonomy in decisions about the management of her pregnancy. An important area for perinatal research is to evaluate these strategies in terms of their enhancement of patient autonomy, reduction of vulnerability, and improvement of the quality of obstetric care for this patient population.

6.6 References

1. McCullough LB, Coverdale JH, Chervenak FA. Ethical challenges of decision making with pregnant patients who have schizophrenia. Am J Obstet Gynecol 2002;187:696–702.
2. American Psychiatric Association. Diagnostic and Statistical Manual of Mental Disorders, 4th ed. Washington, DC: American Psychiatric Association, 1994.
3. American Psychiatric Association. Practice guidelines for the treatment of patients with schizophrenia. Am J Psych 1997;194:supplement.
4. Miller LJ, Finnerty M. Sexuality, pregnancy and childrearing among women with schizophrenia spectrum disorders. Psychiatr Serv 1996;47:502–506.
5. Knutsen E, DuRard C. Previously unrecognized physical illnesses in psychotic patients. Hosp Com Psych 1991;42:182–186.
6. Sacks M, Dermatis H, Looser-Ott S, Burton W, Perry S. Undetected HIV infection among acutely ill psychotic inpatients. Am J Psych 1992;149:544–545.
7. Coverdale JH, Turbott S, Roberts H. Family planning needs and STD risk behaviors of female psychiatric outpatients. Brit J Psych 1997;171:69–72.
8. Coverdale JH, Turbott S. Sexual and physical abuse of chronically ill psychiatric outpatients compared with a matched sample of medical outpatients. J Nerv Ment Disease 2000;188:440–445.

9. Speilvogel A, Vile J. Treatment and outcomes of psychotic patients during pregnancy and childbirth. Birth 1992;19:131–137.
10. Sacker A, Done DJ, Crow TJ. Obstetric complications in children born to parents with schizophrenia: a meta-analysis of case-control studies. Psychol Med 1996;26:279–287.
11. Jablensky A, Zubrick S, Morgan V, Bower C, Pinder T. The offspring of women with schizophrenia and affective psychoses: a population study. Schizophrenia Res 2000;41:8.
12. Bennedsen BE, Mortensen PB, Olesen AV, Henriksen TB. Congenital malformations, stillbirths, and infant deaths among children of women with schizophrenia. Arch Gen Psych 2001;58:674–679.
13. Coverdale J, Aruffo J. Family planning needs of female chronic psychiatric outpatients. Am J Psychiatry 1989;146:1489–1491.
14. Regier DA, Farmer ME, Rae DS, Locke BZ, Keith SJ, Judd LL, Goodwin FK. Comorbidity of mental disorders with alcohol and other drug abuse: results from the epidemiologic catchment area (ECA) study. JAMA 264:2511–2518,1990.
15. Miller LJ. Sexuality, reproduction and family planning in women with schizophrenia. Schizophrenia Bull, 23:623–635,1997.
16. Coverdale J, Falloon IRH, Turbott SH. Sexually transmitted disease and family planning counseling of psychiatric patients in New Zealand. Australia New Zealand J Psychiatry, 31:285–290,1997.
17. McLennan JD, Garguli R. Family planning and parenthood needs of women with severe mental illness: clinicians' perspective. Comm Ment Health J 1999;35:369–380.
18. Miller LJ. Psychotic denial of pregnancy: phenomenology and clinical management. Hosp Comm Psych 1990;41:1233–1237.
19. McCullough LB, Chervenak FA. Ethics in Obstetrics and Gynecology. New York: Oxford University Press, 1994.
20. McCullough LB, Coverdale JH, Bayer T, Chervenak FA. Ethically justified guidelines for family planning interventions to prevent pregnancy with female chronic mental patients. Am J Obstet Gynecol 1992;167:19–25.
21. Coverdale JH, Chervenak FA, McCullough LB, Bayer T. Ethically justified clinically comprehensive guidelines for the management of the depressed pregnant patient. Am J Obstet Gynecol 1996;171:169–173.
22. White BC. Competence to Consent. Washington, DC: Georgetown University Press, 1994.
23. Grisso T, Appelbaum PS. Assessing Competency to Consent to Treatment: A Guide for Physicians and other Health Professionals. New York: Oxford University Press, 1998.
24. Faden RR, Beauchamp TL. A History and Theory of Informed Consent. New York: Oxford University Press, 1986.
25. Altschuler LL, Cohen L, Szuba MP, Burt VK, Gitlin M, Mintz J. Pharmacologic management of psychiatric illness during pregnancy: dilemmas and guidelines. Am J Psychiatry 1996;153:592–606.
26. Falloon IRH, Held T, Roncone R, Coverdale JH, Laidlaw T. Optimal treatment strategies to enhance recovery from schizophrenia. Aust N Z J Psychiatry 1998;32:43–49.
27. McCullough LB, Wilson NL, Teasdale TA, Kolpakchi AL, Skelly J. Mapping personal, familial, and professional values in long-term care decisions. Gerontologist 1993;33:324–332.
28. Buchanan AE, Brock DW. Deciding for Others: The Ethics of Surrogate Decision Making. Cambridge: Cambridge University Press, 1989.
29. Jacobsen T, Miller LJ. Mentally ill mothers who have killed: three cases addressing the issue of future parenting capability. Psychiatr Serv 1998;49:650–657.
30. Jacobson T, Miller NJ, Kirkwood K. Assessing parenting capacity in individuals with severe mental illness: a comprehensive service. J Ment Health Admin 1997;24:189–199.
31. Steadman HJ, Monahan J, Appelbaum PS, Grisso T, Mulvey EP, Roth LH, Robbins PC, Klassen D. Designing a new generation of risk assessment research. In Violence and Mental Disorders:

Developments in Risk Assessment, Monahan J, Steadman HJ, eds. Chicago: University of Chicago Press, 1994.
32. Chervenak FA, McCullough LB, Skupski DW. An ethical justification for emergency, coerced cesarean delivery. Obstet Gynecol 1993;82:1029–1035.

6.7 Summary points

- The perinatologist should recognize and address the distinctive ethical challenges created by chronically and variably impaired capacity for autonomous decision making by pregnant patients with major mental disorders.
- To the degree clinically practicable, the perinatologist should attempt assisted decision making with pregnant patients with major mental disorders.
- When assisted decision making is not clinically practicable, the perinatologist should lead a surrogate decision making process, guided by the substituted judgment and best interests standards.
- A Ulysses contract is a powerful preventive ethics tool for advance decision making with pregnant patients with major mental disorders.

7 Neonatal management

7.1 Introduction

Perinatal ethics includes both obstetric ethics and neonatal ethics. Previous chapters have explored major topics in the ethical obligations of the perinatologist to the pregnant and fetal patient. In this chapter, we address the perinatologist's ethical obligations to the neonatal patient. We begin with an explanation of the sharp contrast between obstetric and neonatal ethics, which together constitute perinatal ethics. We then explore the implications of neonatal ethics for justified limits on resuscitation and neonatal critical and for the perinatologist's professional responsibility to reject infanticide, with explicit reference to the Groningen Protocol.[1]

7.2 Neonatal medical ethics: Delivery makes a difference

In the professional responsibility model of perinatal ethics, delivery of a live born child makes a difference. Before delivery, the perinatologist's ethical obligations to the fetal patient are beneficence-based and must, in all cases, be balanced against the perinatologist's beneficence-based and autonomy-based obligations to the pregnant patient. In the professional responsibility model of perinatal ethics, the perinatologist's ethical obligations after delivery are owed to the neonatal patient and are also beneficence-based. The perinatologist has ethical obligations to the parents of the newborn but not because they are the perinatologist's patient; the newborn is. The perinatologist has autonomy-based obligations to the parents in their role as surrogate decision maker for their child, who is a patient. However, parental autonomy is constrained by the parents' beneficence-based obligations to their child, who is a patient.

The beneficence-based obligations of the perinatologist and parents to a child, who is a patient, originate in the best interests of the child standard, one of the core concepts of pediatric ethics.[2] The best interests of the child standard requires healthcare professionals to protect and promote the health-related interests of pediatric patients. The clinical ethical judgment about what should count as the best interests of the pediatric patient focuses on the patient; the patient's parents' interests are not included because they are not the pediatric healthcare professional's patient. Like all patients, the best interests of the pediatric patient should be understood biopsychosocially, a concept introduced by George Engel.[3–6] Such an approach prevents biomedical reductionism and consequent, excessively narrow, and therefore clinically inadequate diagnostic and therapeutic reasoning. The perinatologist is competent to protect and promote the health-related interests of the child: the prevention of mortality and morbidity, as well as pain, distress, and suffering that are not necessary in order to prevent mortality and morbidity. The obligation to prevent mortality is not absolute, an obligation to preserve life at all costs, which is known as vitalism. Instead, the obligation to preserve life is limited: not every incremental reduction of mortality is worth the increase morbidity, pain, distress, and suffering and the decreased developmental capacity that they cause in the outcomes of resuscitation and neonatal critical care.

Parents are bound by beneficence-based obligations to protect and promote the health-related interests of their child, who is a patient.[2] The parents' beneficence-based obligations are a function of, and therefore directly parallel, the perinatologist's. The ethical logic of such beneficence-based obligations is that they constrain parental autonomy. Parental authority to make decisions on their child's clinical care is a direct function of parents' fulfilling their beneficence-based obligation to authorize clinical management that is reliably expected to clinically benefit their child. In particular, parents have a beneficence-based obligation to authorize effective treatment for the clinical management of life-threatening and other conditions in their child. In the United States, this ethical obligation may be enforced by court orders and referral to Child Protective Services.

There is another sharp contrast between obstetric ethics and neonatal ethics. In obstetric ethics, the pregnant woman is the ultimate decision maker. Her husband or partner surely has a stake in the outcome of her pregnancy, but that individual is not the decision maker. The pregnant woman is, therefore, free to take account of her husband's or partner's beliefs and preferences as the pregnant woman determines for herself. In pediatric ethics, both parents share decision-making authority over their child. Together, they act as their child's surrogate decision makers. Inasmuch as the neonate does not yet have beliefs and preferences, the substituted judgment standard (which requires surrogate decision makers, as reliably as they can, to make decisions reflective of what the patient would have decided) does not apply. The best interests standard (which requires the surrogate decision makers, as reliably as they can, to make decisions that protect and promote the health-related interests of the patient) does. This explains further why parental autonomy is exercised under the constraint of the best interests of the child standard.

7.3 Justified limits on resuscitation and neonatal critical care

Neonatal critical care often begins with resuscitation in the delivery room. Critical care has a short-term goal, the prevention of the imminent death of the patient. Critical care also has a long-term goal, survival with an acceptable outcome. An acceptable outcome can be understood from a clinical perspective: the patient survives with at least some interactive capacity that will allow for subsequent cognitive and motor development. Perinatal ethics is not vitalist, i.e. perinatal ethics does not endorse the view that mere survival, survival with irreversible loss of interactive capacity or "life at all costs," is an acceptable outcome from a clinical perspective. An acceptable outcome can also be understood from the patient's perspective: the remaining interactive capacity results in the patient remaining able to engage in valued life tasks and to derive satisfaction from doing so. When this is the case, the patient has an acceptable quality of life.

We emphasize that this quality-of-life perspective on an acceptable outcome does not apply to neonates, for three compelling reasons. While neonates have distinct personalities and surely have developmental tasks, they do not yet have the cognitive and affective capacity to identify and commit to valued life tasks and make the biopsychosocially sophisticated judgment that engaging in valued life tasks results in sufficient satisfaction. In addition, studies that compare self-reported quality of life of children with disabilities compared to non-disabled controls show no difference.[7] Finally, physicians' judgments of the quality of life of patients with major illness or disability are lower than self-reported judgments of quality of life by patients themselves.[8]

As a result, an acceptable outcome for a neonate from resuscitation and critical care should be understood to be beneficence-based. In the discourse of pediatric ethics, judgments about outcomes should be guided by the best interests of the child standard. On the basis of this standard, the perinatologist should identify the medically reasonable alternatives for managing the neonate's condition.

Resuscitation and neonatal critical care should be understood as trials of intervention: they should be undertaken and continued as long as it is reasonable in beneficence-based, deliberative clinical ethical judgment to expect that the short-term and long-term outcomes will be achieved. When this is not the case, resuscitation is justifiably considered futile. Blackhall, in a landmark article on the futility of cardiopulmonary resuscitation, set the threshold for futility appropriately high: the expected failure rate should range from 97–100 %.[9] The ethical justification for this conservative approach is that it errs on the side of caution, which clinicians should do when the life of a patient is at stake.

This general meaning of futility, however, lacks clinical utility, because it is clinically not fine-grained. Clinically fine-grained and clinically applicable concepts of futility can be identified. We now specify three such concepts that apply in neonatal resuscitation and critical care.[10]

The first is physiologic futility and applies to both resuscitation and critical care. This concept applies when, in beneficence-based, deliberative clinical ethical judgment, it is not reasonable to expect the physiologic outcome of a clinical intervention to occur. When this is the case, it is not reasonable to expect that the short-term goal of resuscitation and critical care will be achieved. To apply this concept clinically, the outcome must be clearly specified. For resuscitation, the physiologic outcome is restoration of spontaneous circulation. Transient heart beats, a physiologic effect of resuscitation, do not count as the physiologic outcome. The physiologic outcome of mechanical ventilation is maintenance of adequate levels of oxygenation of the patient's organs and tissues. When in beneficence-based, deliberative clinical ethical judgment, it is not reasonable to expect that the clearly specified outcome of a clinical intervention will occur, the obligation to provide it does not exist. If resuscitation has not been initiated and can reliably be judged prospectively to be physiologically futile, then the perinatologist should recommend that it not be initiated. If resuscitation has been initiated as a trial and becomes physiologically futile, then the perinatologist should discontinue it. If subsequent neonatal critical care has been initiated as a trial and becomes physiologically futile, the perinatologist should recommend that it be discontinued.

The second is imminent-demise futility. This concept does not apply to resuscitation but does apply to critical care after it has been initiated as a trial of intervention. This concept applies when, in beneficence-based, deliberative clinical ethical judgment, the patient is expected to die during the current admission and never recover interactive capacity before death occurs. When this is the case, it is not reasonable to expect that the short-term goal critical care will be achieved. When in beneficence-based, deliberative clinical ethical judgment, it is not reasonable to expect that the child will survive and that death will occur before interactive capacity is recovered, the obligation to provide continued critical care does not exist. When neonatal critical care becomes imminent-demise futile, the perinatologist should recommend that it be discontinued.

The third is clinical or overall futility. This concept does not apply to resuscitation but does apply to critical care after it has been initiated as a trial of intervention. This concept applies when, in beneficence-based, deliberative clinical ethical judgment, the patient is expected to survive but never recover interactive capacity. When this is the case, it is reasonable to expect that the short-term goal critical care, understood from a clinical perspective, will be achieved but it is not reasonable to expect that the long-term goal of critical care will be achieved. When in beneficence-based, deliberative clinical ethical judgment, it is not reasonable to expect that the child will recover interactive capacity, the obligation to provide continued critical care does not exist. When neonatal critical care becomes overall or clinically futile, the perinatologist should recommend that it be discontinued.

In adult critical care, quality-of-life futility applies when the patient is expected to survive (the short-term goal is achieved) and retain at last some interactive capacity (the long-term goal from a clinical perspective is achieved) but not support the patient in pursuing valued life tasks or in gaining sufficient satisfaction from the patient's perspective from doing so (the long-term goal from the patient's perspective is not achieved). For the reasons explained above, quality-of-life futility has no application in the neonatal component of perinatal ethics.

Conveying the concept of resuscitation and neonatal critical care as trials of intervention to prospective parents before delivery, when the perinatologist should be concerned about the limits of resuscitation and neonatal critical care, is a crucial first step in a preventive ethics approach to the clinical application of these three specified concepts of futility. Conveying this concept prepares them for the challenging conversation that will occur when one or more of the above three specified concepts of futility apply.

Neonatal critical care may also be foregone or discontinued in the United States under applicable advance directives legislation. These statutes typically allow for both non-initiation and discontinuation of life-sustaining treatment, which includes essentially all of neonatal critical care, when the pediatric (or adult) patient has been diagnosed with a terminal or irreversible condition, as these are defined in the statute. These statutes also, typically, provide for immunity from criminal and civil liability when a patient is allowed to die under the provisions of the statute.

Parents will respond differently and often at a different pace to the perinatologist's recommendation that neonatal critical care be discontinued. The perinatologist has the professional responsibility to engage the appropriate social and spiritual support for parents as they face the calamity of their child's death. Hospitals should combine the resources of palliative care, social work, ethics consultation, and, for parents who are members of faith communities or those who request it, chaplaincy to support parents. The goal should be to help parents understand that loving their child is compatible with accepting limits on the capacity of excellent medical and nursing care to alter outcomes when one or more of the three specified concepts of futility apply.

7.4 The perinatologist's professional responsibility to reject infanticide: The Groningen Protocol is clinically unnecessary, unscientific, and unprofessional

The Groningen Protocol was introduced in 2005, in the *New England Journal of Medicine*.[11] The Protocol provides for "deliberate life-ending procedures" for infants with a "hopeless prognosis" and "unbearable suffering" when specific requirements are met. The requirements are the following: "the diagnosis and prognosis must be certain; hopeless and unbearable suffering must be present; the diagnosis, prognosis, and unbearable suffering must be confirmed by at least one independent doctor; both parents must give informed consent; the procedure must be performed in accordance with the accepted medical standard."[11] The Protocol is not intended for infants "with no chance of survival," because the accepted standard of care for such patients is non-intervention. Nor is the Protocol intended for infants with "very poor prognosis ... dependent on intensive care,"[11] because non-intervention for such patients can be ethically justified. The Protocol was approved and adopted by the Dutch Association of Paediatrics in 2005.[12]

The authors of the protocol have published one report on the implementation of the Protocol in which euthanasia was performed in twenty-two cases of "severe suffering without hope of improvement," twenty-one of which were cases of spina bifida.[13] The clinical criteria invoked to support ending the lives of these twenty-two patients were "poor quality of life, predicted lack of self-sufficiency, predicted inability to communicate, expected hospital dependency, and long life expectancy" of burden.[11]

Since the Protocol was published, there has been an active discussion regarding its appropriateness.[1,12,14–26] We now address three questions: Is the Protocol clinically necessary?; Is the Protocol scientific?; Is the Protocol professional?

7.4.1 Is The Groningen Protocol clinically necessary?

The patient population for which the Protocol is intended to provide clinical guidance is infants with a "hopeless prognosis" and "unbearable suffering." There is already an ethically accepted standard of care for such infants: withholding or discontinuing life-sustaining treatment and providing hospice and palliative care.[27,28] The ethical argument in support of this standard is beneficence-based: when one or more of the above clinical ethical concepts of futility apply or when the patient is diagnosed with a terminal or irreversible condition. These justifications become even stronger when the disease-related and iatrogenic burden of morbidity, pain, distress, and suffering is increasing. In such cases, the alleviation of pain, distress, and suffering, and the prevention of further morbidity becomes paramount and should guide beneficence-based clinical judgment and decision making. In such circumstances, physicians should recommend that life-sustaining treatment be discontinued and be replaced with appropriate palliation and hospice care.

Rob de Jong succinctly answers our first question: "When such a newborn is not treated, modern palliative care always will suffice in eliminating possible discomfort. There is no reason whatsoever for active life-termination of these newborns."[12] Moreover, parental "requests to hasten death are generally abandoned" when "competent and compassionate palliative care, including the use of adequate analgesia and sedation for the treatment of rapidly progressive symptoms"[12] is provided.

Not only is the Protocol clinically unnecessary, it was clinically misdirected. Induced abortion, when a fetal anomaly such as spina bifida is present, is legally permitted in most jurisdictions in most developed countries, including the Netherlands, and has strong ethical support. In Chapter 2, we show that the ethics of induced abortion in such cases is autonomy-based: the pregnant woman is free to withhold or withdraw the moral status of being a patient from the previable fetus. When the pregnant woman does so, termination of pregnancy does not involve the killing of a patient and is, therefore, permissible in the professional responsibility model of perinatal ethics, as we explain in Chapter 2.[29] With a technology utilized throughout the developed world, modern ultrasound screening, spina bifida can be diagnosed before viability. Instead of bringing forward a controversial and clinically unnecessary protocol, efforts should have been sooner directed toward making modern ultrasound screening to all pregnant women in the Netherlands. Fortunately, "new regulations providing access for all pregnant women became effective in January 2007."[20] This has had the unsurprising effect of eliminating cases in which the Protocol was applied: "Recently, the multidisciplinary review committee for newborn euthanasia, installed in March 2007, announced that no euthanasia cases were reported in the Netherlands in the past year."[20]

7.4.2 Is the Groningen Protocol scientific?

A clinical protocol, to be scientifically valid, must provide the nature and level of evidence for its components. The chief components of the Groningen Protocol are unbearable suffering and the four clinical criteria of "poor quality of life, predicted lack of self-sufficiency, predicted inability to communicate, expected hospital dependency, and long life expectancy" of burden.[11]

Unbearable suffering. Unbearable suffering occurs when a patient is in severe acute or chronic pain that cannot be relieved. Evidence-based reasoning requires that, to validate this criterion, a literature review is necessary as the first step. We performed a literature review using "spina bifida" and "suffering," which yielded 120 citations, with 99 published in 2004 or earlier.[30] We used this cut-off to identify articles that were available to the authors of the Protocol prior to its publication in 2005. None of these are cited in the Protocol and none document serious suffering in children with spina bifida.

Rob de Jong has undertaken the first and most comprehensive review of the scientific evidence for the clinical application of the Protocol. Rob de Jong reports that "not any convincing evidence can be found in the literature that newborns with MMC [meningomyeocele] actually do suffer from intractable pain in the days after birth caused by their back lesion or by other complications."[12] Concerning chronic pain in infants with spina bifida, "the notion of 'unbearable and hopeless suffering' is never mentioned" in any of the papers Rob de Jong reviewed.[12] The Protocol's failure to review the relevant scientific literature concerning short-term and long-term unbearable suffering from spina bifida and the lack of a provision of an objective evidence base that such suffering exists in infants with spina bifida make it unscientific to invoke unbearable suffering. The Protocol is a failure in this respect.

Poor quality of life. Quality of life is a concept without a fixed definition in medical literature.[1] It should be understood to mean engaging in valued life tasks and deriving sufficient satisfaction from doing so. Evidence-based reason requires that, to validate this criterion, a literature review is necessary as the first step. We performed a literature review using "spina bifida" and "quality of life," which yielded 175 citations, with 125 published in 2004 or earlier.[31] The Protocol cites none of these articles.

There are many challenges in using quality of life assessment by others than the individual affected. It is generally accepted that the best standard for assessing quality of life is self-reported quality of life.[7,32] The self-reported quality of life of children, adolescents, and adults with spina bifida and also those who were born extremely prematurely displays wide variation. Saigal and Tyson, in a comprehensive literature review, identify the major implication of this wide variation: "*What is clear is that having a biological impairment does not automatically translate in a poor self-assessed quality of life.*"[7] It directly follows that the premise of the Protocol, that two independent physicians (or even a multidisciplinary team) can predict future quality of life is scientifically invalid. The Protocol's failure to review the relevant scientific literature concerning self-reported quality of life of children with spina bifida and the lack of a provision of an objective evidence base that self-reported quality of life is unacceptable. It is unscientific to invoke quality of life. The Protocol is a failure in this respect.

Predicted lack of self-sufficiency. Rob de Jong reviewed reports on long-term follow-up of patients with spina bifida.[12] There is wide variation in the level of independence in this patient population, which calls into question the evidence-base for the Protocol's use of this criterion. Nowhere does the Protocol provide a literature review or a critical analysis of this subject. The result is that this criterion is vague, with important ethical implications that we address in the next section. While it is clear that spina bifida results in disability, to use predicted lack of self-sufficiency requires an evidence base concerning its clinical variation and impact on development. The Protocol's failure to review the relevant scientific literature concerning predicted lack of self-sufficiency from spina bifida and the lack of a provision of an objective evidence base about the variation and impact of disability from spina bifida make it unscientific to invoke predicted lack of self-sufficiency. The Protocol is a failure in this respect.

Predicted inability to communicate. Rob de Jong reports that in the Dutch article on the case series in which the Protocol was applied, for 18 of the 22 cases, "future communication of and with the child would not be possible, neither verbally or nonverbally."[12] Rob de Jong correctly points out that for this outcome to occur, the patients would have to be "in a deep coma or in a persistent vegetative state," neither of which is "applicable to a newborn with MMC and hydrocephalus."[12] Rob de Jong quotes from a 1984 article by John Freeman: "Virtually all infants with spina bifida are capable of meaningful human relationships, independent of the lesion. Indeed, most are of normal intelligence."[12,33] Advances in the treatment of spina bifida in the past two decades only reinforce this conclusion. The Protocol's failure to review the relevant scientific literature concerning predicted inability to communicate and the lack of a provision of an objective evidence base about the variation and impact of this alleged inability make it unscientific to invoke predicted inability to communicate. The Protocol is a failure in this respect.

Expected hospital dependency. Rob de Jong reports no evidence to support the claim that patients with spina bifida will have an unusually large number of hospitalizations, "compared to persons with other congenital malformations or congenital diseases or some acquired diseases."[12] Rob de Jong concludes that: "It seems hardly possible to quantify this criterion in such a way that it can be used to justify life termination of vital newborns."[12] The Protocol provides no evidence base that might respond to this conclusion. The Protocol's failure to review the relevant scientific literature concerning expected hospital dependency and the lack of a provision of an objective evidence base about the variation and impact of hospitalizations make it unscientific to invoke expected hospital dependency. The Protocol is a failure in this respect.

Long life expectancy of burden. Rob de Jong points out that patients with spina bifida experience most of their hospitalizations in the first two decades of life, with hospitalizations "decreasing when they grow older and when disabilities and coping with these disabilities are gradually stabilized."[12] There is, therefore, no evidence of a life-time of unbearable suffering based on a life expectancy of burden. The Protocol's failure to review the relevant scientific literature concerning long life expectancy of burden from spina bifida and the lack of a provision of an objective evidence base about the variation and impact of such alleged burden make it unscientific to invoke unbearable suffering. The Protocol is a failure in this respect. In all of its key scientific concepts the Protocol is a systematic failure.

7.4.3 Is the Groningen Protocol professional?

A clinical protocol that concerns deliberate life-ending procedures must also provide an ethical justification for its components if it is to be compatible with the professional model of perinatal ethics. The chief components of the Groningen Protocol are unbearable suffering and the four clinical criteria of "poor quality of life, predicted lack of self-sufficiency, predicted inability to communicate, expected hospital dependency, and long life expectancy" of burden.[11] In addition, the Protocol emphasizes the need for transparency.[11]

Ethics is not a matter of personal opinion but reasoned argument. There are standards for argument-based ethics that can be used to evaluate whether the Protocol is ethical. The most fundamental requirement of argument-based ethics is that concepts used in ethical reasoning be explained clearly and used consistently' as explained in Chapters 1 and 10.

Unbearable suffering. Suffering should be carefully distinguished from pain and distress. Pain is a report in the central nervous system of tissue damage, accompanied by awareness. Distress is a disruption of an individual's normal or usual behavioral repertoire. Suffering is a complex biopsychosocial phenomenon in which an individual experiences limitations on the pursuit and/or achievement of desired goals.

Unbearable suffering was defined clearly by one of the founders of bioethics, Richard McCormick, in a landmark article in the *Journal of the American Medical Association* in 1974. McCormick explained that sometimes disease-related and iatrogenic morbidity and disability can overwhelm an individual, such that he or she is reduced to a state in which he or she experiences only the struggle to survive.[34] When pain or distress also occur for patients only struggling to survive, suffering becomes even more unbearable, because the individual no longer gains anything clinically or personally from experiencing pain and distress. None of this applies clinically to infants with spina bifida.

Nowhere does the Protocol clearly define "suffering," much less "unbearable suffering." It is impossible to construct a valid argument in ethics when such crucial concepts are left systematically vague.

A recent defense of the Groningen Protocol has not changed this judgment. Lindemann and Verkerk claim that unbearable suffering has "a perfectly ordinary, everyday meaning," which they then do not articulate.[19] This simply reinforces the systematic vagueness of the concept. Because of this systematic vagueness, it is unethical to use the concept of unbearable suffering as utilized in the Protocol. The Protocol is a failure in this respect.

Poor quality of life. In the Protocol, the concept of quality of life is never explicitly defined. The Protocol fails to recognize that the concept of quality of life does not apply to infants, as explained above. The Protocol does assert criteria purported to be relevant to quality of life judgments. The Protocol relies on two physicians or the healthcare team to make this judgment.

This procedural requirement assumes that physicians' judgments about quality of life are reliable. In their systematic review, Saigal and Tyson report that studies show that "proxy respondents tend to report higher morbidity and lower QoL [quality of life] than the individuals whose perceived health status and QoL is being judged."[7] Nowhere does the Protocol acknowledge this potential bias in physicians' judgments about future quality of life or explain how the requirement of having two physicians or a healthcare team make such judgments responsibly manage this potential bias.

The Protocol calls for the consent of parents, based, in part, on their assessment of their child's future quality of life. Saigal and Tyson report that parental judgments of quality of life "may be negatively influenced by the burden of caregiving, stress, and their own mental, social, and economic status."[7] Nowhere does the Protocol acknowledge this potential bias or propose a strategy for responsibly managing it.

Defenders of the Protocol claim that parents are "uniquely qualified to judge what quality of life the [newborn] child would find acceptable."[19] In response, Daniel Callahan, another founder of the field of bioethics, states: "That will come as news to most parents who, looking at their newborn child, will be surprised to learn that they have such notable powers of discernment."[21]

Saigal and Tyson consider self-reported quality of life, its most reliable measure. Their review of the literature on the self-reported quality of life of individuals who are survivors of neonatal care leads them to conclude that "*having a biological impairment does not automatically translate in a poor self-assessed quality of life.*"[7] It follows directly that, even if physicians or parents were, contrary to fact, *reliable* predictors of future quality of life of children with spina bifida or other disabling conditions, they could not make accurate predictions because there is no stable relationship between future biological impairment and future quality of life. Because there is, therefore, no scientific foundation for predictive judgments of quality of life by physicians or parents, it is unethical to use the concept of quality of life to make such predictions as called for in the Protocol. The Protocol is a failure in this respect.

Predicted lack of self-sufficiency. The Protocol makes the implicit assumption that dependence on others is an ethically inferior condition. Relying on implicit assumptions violates the standards of argument-based ethics (see Chapter 10), because implicit assumptions are not clearly stated, creating an increased risk that conclusions drawn from implicit assumptions will not be valid.

Rob de Jong makes a counter-argument: "Most people who do live a meaningful life are dependent on others or interdependent on each other. In fact, interdependency and especially the willingness to care for other (perhaps dependent) people can be considered as a criterion of a truly civilized society."[12] The internationally prominent American political philosopher, John Rawls (1921–2002), formalized this idea in his theory of justice. A just society provides fair equality of opportunity for human advancement, especially for those who are most vulnerable. Benefitting those who are least well off in virtue of physical, psychological, or social vulnerability is a requirement of justice in societies with economic resources,[35] i.e. the developed world, including the Netherlands. Amartya Sen has argued that justice requires societies to shoulder the burdens of those with disabilities.[36] Argument-based ethics requires that any claim that dependence is ethically inferior satisfactorily rebut these powerful ethical arguments to the contrary (see Chapter 10). The failure to meet this requirement of argument-based ethics means that it is unethical to use the concept of dependence as utilized in the Protocol. The Protocol is a failure in this respect.

Predicted inability to communicate. Argument-based ethics requires that ethical concepts be clinically applicable. The Protocol never clearly explains the concept of inability to communicate. Rob de Jong correctly points out that this criterion applies to patients in deep coma or persistent vegetative state.[12] Neither of these states is relevant to spina bifida. This means that the criterion of predicted inability to communicate does not have clinical application to the patient population to which the Protocol has been applied. The failure to meet the requirement of clinical applicability means that it is unethical to use the concept of inability to communicate as utilized in the Protocol. The Protocol is a failure in this respect.

Long life expectancy of burden. The use of this criterion in the Protocol cannot be separated from the criterion of unbearable suffering. This is because all chronic conditions, including not just spina bifida but the common chronic diseases of aging, involve biopsychosocial burden, and therefore the potential for suffering of varying and unpredictable degrees. Such suffering is ethically significant and should be addressed in the care of patients with chronic diseases and conditions, a recognized standard of care for chronic diseases and conditions. By itself, the criterion of long life expectancy of burden does not ethically justify non-treatment, much less the deliberate ending of life as called for in the Protocol. To reach this conclusion, unbearable suffering must also be invoked, but we argued above that it is unethical to do so. The Protocol is a failure in this respect.

Parental consent, parental responsibility, and co-fiduciary responsibility of physicians and parents. In the professional responsibility model of perinatal ethics, the physician is the fiduciary of the patient, including the newborn and child. Fulfilling the three commitments for becoming a professional physician – to becoming scientifically and clinically competent, to the protection and promotion of the patient's health-related and other interests as the physician's primary concern and motivation and to keeping self-interest systematically secondary, and to maintaining, strengthening, and passing on medicine as a public trust for the benefit of future physicians, patients, and society (see Chapter 1) – places the beneficence-based interests of the patient, the best interests of the child, in trust to the perinatologist for their safe-keeping and protection. The same is true for parents of a child who becomes a patient; they become the fiduciaries of their child, who is a patient. Parents are expected to be competent in the general skills of parenting and to put the interests of their children ahead of their own, within reasonable limits of self-sacrifice. Parental authority over their children is a function of their fulfilling their fiduciary role. Failure to do so provides the ethical justification for laws prohibiting child abuse and neglect. Thus, the rights of parents to make decisions about the medical care of their children are a function of the parents fulfilling their fiduciary role. Parental rights are not independent of their fiduciary role. In their fiduciary role, parents are ethically obligated to authorize medical care that is reliably expected to protect and promote the health-related and other interests of their child, as required by the best interests of the child standard. Parents are not free to authorize medical intervention that does not meet this ethical requirement. As a consequence, the American Academic of Pediatrics invokes the concept of parental permission for medically indicated treatment of children, not parental consent, because the concept of consent would allow parents to refuse needed medical treatment of a child.[2] Adults are free to refuse such treatment for themselves, but not for children to whom they owe a fiduciary obligation of protection.

Parents' fulfillment of their fiduciary role in the medical care of their children is a function of evidence-based clinical judgment of physicians about which clinical interventions are reliably expected to protect and promote the health-related and other interests of their child. In the medical setting, therefore, physicians and parents are co-fiduciaries of pediatric patients.

The ethical concept of co-fiduciary responsibility of physicians and parents in pediatrics has direct implications for the Groningen Protocol. The fulfillment of parental fiduciary responsibilities in the medical setting is dependent on physicians' fulfillment of their fiduciary responsibilities. The component of physicians' fiduciary role most relevant here is scientific and clinical competence. The systematic violation of scientific and ethical standards for valid clinical protocols by the Groningen Protocol means that no physician can, consistent with fiduciary responsibility to a neonatal patient, apply the Protocol in clinical practice. Nor can any physician with ethical justification offer or recommend the clinical implementation of the Protocol to parents. Finally, no parent can with ethical justification authorize the clinical application of the Protocol.

In their case series report, the authors of the Groningen Protocol report that in 4 of the 22 cases was the request for deliberate ending of life initiated by the parents, a violation of the parents' fiduciary role.[13] Presumably, in the remaining 18 cases, the physician offered or recommended the Protocol, a violation of the physician's professional role.

The Protocol calls for parental consent. Kodish has criticized this requirement because it invokes the wrong ethical concept, when the correct concept is parental permission.[18] For this reason alone, the procedural requirement of parental consent in the Protocol is ethically inappropriate. In addition, the concept of parents' co-fiduciary responsibility in the medical setting means that giving permission to implement the Protocol is unethical. There is, therefore, no ethically meaningful role for parents other than to appropriately assert their fiduciary responsibility and reject physicians' unethical offers or recommendations of the Protocol. The Protocol is a failure in this respect.

Accepted medical standard. The Protocol's implicit assumption that there is an "accepted medical standard" for doing something, deliberately ending the life of patients unnecessarily and without any scientific, clinical, or ethical justification, is egregiously antithetical to physicians' professional, fiduciary responsibility to patients. Kodish, a leader in pediatric ethics, succinctly states the ethical implication of the physician's fiduciary responsibility regarding the Protocol: "Stop killing babies."[18] The Protocol is a failure in this respect.

Transparency. The Protocol calls for transparency, i.e. the routine reporting of cases of infant euthanasia to the appropriate authorities.[11,20] This is important, because such clinically and ethically significant actions should not be secret. The Protocol, however, misunderstands the ethical nature and importance of transparency. Transparency is an essential component of accountability for the competent and ethical practice of medicine, making accountability an essential component of fiduciary responsibility.[37,38] In other words, physicians should accept a requirement of transparency for fulfilling their fiduciary obligations to their patients. Euthanasia of newborns violates fiduciary responsibility and is, therefore, unethical. Being transparent about unethical clinical practices does not make those practices ethical. Ironically, the Groningen Protocol's requirement of transparency and its publication in *The New England Journal of Medicine*[11] have done the unintended professional and public service of exposing the unethical killing of infants in the Netherlands. The Protocol is a failure in this respect.

Cultural relativism. Some defenders of the Protocol have claimed that: "Concerning the larger question of whether the practice for which the protocol was developed can be morally justified, we think it can – in the Netherlands, at any rate."[19] This is the assertion of cultural relativism, which is the view that ethical concepts and arguments cannot meaningfully transcend cultural and national boundaries.

Cultural relativism does not have a place in setting the standards of professional perinatal ethics, because in the professional responsibility model of perinatal ethics, the professional, fiduciary responsibility of perinatologists is transcultural, transnational, and transreligious. As explained in Chapter 1, the concept of professional responsibility originated in Great Britain more than two centuries ago. In the intervening time, this ethical concept has been embraced and made definitive of being a professional in medicine all around the world. The most recent expression of the international reach of medical professionalism can be found in the Physician's Charter,[38] which has been adopted by medical societies throughout the world. In addition, international statements of physicians in many aspects of patient care reflect the transcultural, transnational, and transreligious nature of modern biomedicine and medical ethics. Asserting Dutch exceptionalism totally lacks scientific and ethical plausibility.

There is another relevant transcultural, transnational, and transreligious concept that is relevant, namely human rights. These include the right to appropriate healthcare, which does not include the deliberate ending of life of neonatal patients. Rob de Jong, therefore, puts it well: "Finally, to date it remains unclear ... why international legislation, international human rights instruments, and international medical recommendations appear not to hold in the Netherlands, especially not in newborns with MMC."[2] The Protocol is a failure in this respect. In all of its key ethical concepts, the Protocol is a systematic failure.

7.5 Conclusion

In the professional responsibility model of perinatal ethics, there are ethically justified limits on neonatal critical care. The clinical ethics concepts of physiologic, imminent-demise, and clinical or overall futility, provide an ethically justified, clinically applicable basis for setting such limits. The Groningen Protocol does not do so; it is a clinical, scientific, and professional failure that has no place in perinatal ethics and should not ever be clinically implemented, much less approved by professional organizations, healthcare organizations, or policy makers. This is true for infanticide under any protocol. We agree with Saugstad, who states: "Neonatologists must be extremely careful not [to] start on the slippery slope ending in the Dutch practice of euthanasia of newborns."[14] We also agree with Kodish when he states: "Paediatricians around the world should condemn the Groningen Protocol, and refuse to take part in or be associated with infanticide."[14] We renew our call for the Dutch Association of Paediatrics to revoke its approval and adoption of the Groningen Protocol.

7.6 References

1. Chervenak FA, McCullough LB, Arabin B. Why the Groningen Protocol should be rejected. Hastings Cent Rep 2006;36:30–33.
2. American Academy of Pediatrics, Committee on Bioethics. Informed consent, parental permission, and assent in pediatrics practice. Pediatrics 1995;95:314–317.
3. Engel G. A unified concept of health and disease. IRE Transactions on Medical Electronics 2009; 10.1109/IRET-ME.1960.5008004. Originally appeared in Perspectives in Biology and Medicine 1960;13:48–57.
4. Engel G. The need for a new medical model: a challenge for biomedicine. Science 1977; 196: 129–136. Reproduced in Holistic Med 1989;4:37–53.
5. Engel G. The clinical application of the biopsychosocial model Am J Psychiatry 1980;137:535–544.
6. Engel G. The biopsychosocial model and medical education. New Engl J Med 1982;306:802–805.
7. Saigal S, Tyson J. Measurement of quality of life of survivors of neonatal intensive care: critique and implications. Semin Perinatol 2008;32:59–66.
8. Leplege A, Hunt S. The problem of quality of life in medicine. JAMA 1997;278:47–50.
9. Blackhall L. Must we always use CPR? New Engl J Med 1987;317:1281–1285.
10. McCullough LB, Jones JW. Postoperative futility: a clinical algorithm for setting limits. Brit J Surg 2001;88:1153–1154.
11. Verhagen E, Saier PJJ. The Groningen Protocol – euthanasia in severely ill newborns. N Engl J Med 2005;352:959–962.
12. Rob de Jong TH. Deliberate termination of life in newborns with spina birifda, a critical reappraisal. Childs Nerv Syst 2008;24:13–28.
13. Verhagen AAE, Sol JJ, Brouwer OF, Sauer PJ. Actieve levens-beendiging bij pasgeborenen in Nederland, Een analyse can alle meldingen van 1997–2004. Ned Tijdschr Geneeskd 2005;149:183–188.
14. Saugstad OD. When newborn infants are bound to die. Acta Paediatr 2005;94:1535–1537.
15. Jotkowitz AB, Glick S. The Groningen Protocol: another perspective. J Med Ethics 2006;32:157–158.
16. Manninen BA. A case for justified non-voluntary active euthanasia: exploring the ethics of the Groningen Protocol. J Med Ethics 2006;32:643–651.
17. Kon AA. Neonatal euthanasia is unsupportable: the Groningen Protocol should be abandoned. Theor Med Bioeth 2007;28:453–463.
18. Kodish E. Paediatric ethics: a repudiation of the Groningen Protocol. Lancet 2008;371:892–893.

19. Lindemann H, Verkerk M. Ending the life of a newborn: the Groningen Protocol. Hastings Cent Rep 2008;38:42–51.
20. Verhagen AAE, Sauer PJ. "Are their babies different from ours?" Dutch culture and the Groningen Protocol. Hastings Cent Rep 2008;38:4.
21. Callahan D. "Are their babies different from ours?" Dutch culture and the Groningen Protocol. Hastings Cent Rep 2008;38:4–6.
22. Chervenak FA, McCullough LB, Arabin B. "Are their babies different from ours?" Dutch culture and the Groningen Protocol. Hastings Cent Rep 2008;38:6.
23. Smith T. "Are their babies different from ours?" Dutch culture and the Groningen Protocol. Hastings Cent Rep 2008;38:6.
24. Goldfarb G. "Are their babies different from ours?" Dutch culture and the Groningen Protocol. Hastings Cent Rep 2008;38:7.
25. Lindemann H, Verkerk M. "Are their babies different from ours?" Dutch culture and the Groningen Protocol. Hastings Cent Rep 2008;38:7–8.
26. Catlin A, Novakovich R. The Groningen Protocol: What is it? How do the Dutch use it? And do we use it here? Pediatr Nurs34:247–251.
27. American Academy of Pediatrics, Committee on Bioethics and Committee on Hospital Care. Palliative care for children. Pediatrics 2000;106:351–357.
28. Breeze AC, Lees CC, Kumar A, Missfelder-Lobos HH, Murdoch EM. Palliative care for prenatally diagnosed lethal fetal abnormalities. Arch Dis Child Fetal Neonatal Ed 2007;92:F56–58.
29. McCullough LB, Chervenak FA. Ethics in Obstetrics and Gynecology. New York: Oxford University Press, 1994.
30. PUBMED search performed February 27, 2014. www.ncbi.nlm.nih.gov/sites/entrez.
31. PUBMED search performed February 27, 2014. www.ncbi.nlm.nih.gov/sites/entrez.
32. Zwicker JG, Harris SR. Quality of life of formerly preterm and very low birth weight infants from preschool to adulthood: a systematic review. Pediatrics 2008;121:e366-e376.
33. Freeman JM. Early management and decision making for the treatment of myelomeningocele: a critique. Pediatrics 1984;73:564–566.
34. McCormick RA. To save or let die: the dilemma of modern medicine. JAMA 1974;229:172–176.
35. Rawls J. A Theory of Justice. Cambridge, Mass. Belknap Press of Harvard University Press, 1971.
36. Sen A. Inequality Reexamined Cambridge, Mass.: Harvard University Press, 1992.
37. McCullough LB. The ethical concept of medicine as a profession: its origins in modern medical ethics and implications for physicians. In Kenny N, Shelton W, eds. Lost Virtue: Professional Character Development in Medical Education. New York: Elsevier, 2006:17–27.
38. ABIM Foundation, American Board of Internal Medicine, ACP-ASIM Foundation, American College of Physicians-American Society of Internal Medicine, European Federation of Internal Medicine. Medical professionalism in the new millennium: a physician charter. Ann Intern Med 2002;136:243–246.

7.7 Summary points

- In the professional responsibility model of perinatal ethics, delivery makes a difference: the perinatologist has obligations to the neonatal patient, based on the best interests of the child standard, which is beneficence-based.
- Neonatal resuscitation and critical care should be understood, and presented to prospective parents and parents, as trials of intervention with a short-term

goal, preventing imminent death, and a long-term goal, survival with an acceptable outcome as understood from a clinical perspective.
- It is ethically permissible to discontinue resuscitation when, in deliberative clinical judgment, it is reliably judged to have become physiologically futile.
- It is ethically permissible to forego or discontinue neonatal critical care when, in deliberative clinical judgment, the neonatal patient is reliably judged to have a terminal condition.
- It is ethically permissible to discontinue neonatal critical care when, in deliberative clinical judgment, neonatal critical care has become physiologically, imminent-demise, or clinically or overall futile.
- The Groningen Protocol in clinically unnecessary, unscientific, and unprofessional. It, and infanticide under any protocol, therefore, should be rejected by perinatologists as a violation of the professional responsibility model of perinatal ethics.

8 Perinatal innovation and research

8.1 Introduction

The professional responsibility model of perinatal ethics provides guidance for the improvement of perinatal care for maternal and fetal benefit. This guidance identifies a sequence from animal models, through planned innovation and early-phase and later-phase clinical investigation of both medical and surgical interventions, to the transition to clinical practice. [1,2]

Both innovation and research on pregnant women to improve their health or to improve the health of the fetus and future child present ethical challenges to clinical investigators, Perinatal Innovation Review Committees (PIRCs, a new concept in perinatal practice that we describe in the next section), Institutional Review Boards (IRBs) and Research Ethics Commttees (RECs), and funding agencies.[1–5] Both innovation and research are now rapidly expanding, underscoring the need for a practical, comprehensive ethical framework that will guide professionally responsible perinatal innovation and research and the professionally responsible introduction of their results into clinical practice. In the absence of such a framework, ethically unjustified research may be done. In addition, important clinical research that otherwise might be done may be postponed or never done at all. The result is that "our ignorance harms mothers and babies,"[3] which is not acceptable health policy and practice.

This chapter deploys the professional responsibility model of perinatal ethics, to create a practical, comprehensive ethical framework for innovation and research designed to improve both the health of pregnant women and the health of fetuses and future children, and the introduction of the results of advances in perinatal interventions into clinical practice.[1,2] First, we distinguish innovation from research and explain their proper scientific, clinical, and ethical relationship. We then draw on current research regulations and statements, especially the relevant sections of the United States Common Rule, which provides detailed guidance for investigators and IRBs/RECs in the design and evaluation of perinatal research protocols. We will identify the central ethical challenge of applying this key section to research to improve the health of pregnant women, fetuses, and future children: making a responsible assessment of the risk-benefit ratio. As research involving pregnant women takes two forms – to improve the health of pregnant women and to improve the health of fetal patients – we identify ethically justified criteria for each separately. We close by identifying ethically justified criteria for responsibly managing the transition from investigation to clinical practice for both forms of research.

8.2 Innovation and research

Innovation and research are both forms of experimentation. A perinatologist performs an experiment when he or she provides clinical management, the outcome of which cannot be reliably predicted. When the experiment is performed for the benefit of the patient, then the perinatologist is engaged in innovation. When the experiment is performed for the purpose of creating generalizable knowledge, then the perinatologist is engaged in research.

In the past, both planned and unplanned innovation occurred, the results of which have been mixed in the history of medicine generally, and specifically in the history of perinatology.[6] In 2008 the Society of University Surgeons (SUS),[7] based on pioneering work by McNeally [8], and by Reitsma and Moreno[9], called for the advent of a new era in medical and surgical innovation: prospective peer-review for the scientific, clinical, and ethical justification of innovation. SUS called for institutional review by Surgical Innovation Committees. Here, we extend this call to perinatal innovation and call for the creation of Perinatal Innovation Review Committees (PIRCs). Clinicians proposing perinatal innovation for maternal or fetal benefit should prepare a written protocol that describes previous experience with animal models or simulation, as well as the reported experience to date in the peer-reviewed literature. The proposer should then make an argument for why the innovation should be judged as potentially promising. The nature of the medical or surgical intervention should be described, as well as its documented and theoretical benefits and risks. The informed consent process should also be described. In all cases, this process must include making clear to the pregnant woman (who is the ultimate decision maker about the clinical management of her pregnancy) that (a) the intervention is experimental in that its outcomes cannot be predicted, (b) that the intervention has been reviewed and approved by the PIRC, and (c) she is not ethically obligated to her fetus and future child to accept the innovation. The protocol should define the outcomes that will be measured and clinically evaluated for potential benefit. PIRC-approved innovation becomes pre-research.

If a PIRC-approved planned innovation is successful, then an important aspect of PIRC-approved innovation as pre-research is that the innovator should consider either additional innovation, with PIRC approval, or transition to early-phase research to assess the efficacy and safety of the intervention. Based on previous animal models and simulation, investigators can also begin with early-phase research. Subsequent phases of research should then follows. If the intervention is shown on balance to be clinically beneficial, i.e. in deliberative, beneficence-based clinical judgment it should be considered medically reasonable. Then a transition should be made to clinical practice.

8.3 Current research regulations

The Council of the International Organization of Medical Societies (CIOMS) defines research: "The term 'research' refers to a class of activity designed to develop or contribute to generalizable knowledge. Generalizable knowledge consists of theories, principles or relationships, or the accumulation of information on which they

Table 8.1: The Common Rule, Title 45 Part 46 of the Code of Federal Regulations (45CFR46), Protection of Human Subjects.

„§ 46.204 Research involving pregnant women or fetuses. Pregnant women or fetuses may be involved in research if all of the following conditions are met:

(a) Where scientifically appropriate, preclinical studies, including studies on pregnant animals, and clinical studies, including studies on nonpregnant women, have been conducted and provide data for assessing potential risks to pregnant women and fetuses;

(b) The risk to the fetus is caused solely by interventions or procedures that hold out the prospect of direct benefit for the woman or the fetus; or, if there is no such prospect of benefit, the risk to the fetus is not greater than minimal, and the purpose of the research is the development of important biomedical knowledge which cannot be obtained by any other means;

(c) Any risk is the least possible for achieving the objectives of the research;

(d) If the research holds out the prospect of direct benefit to the pregnant woman, the prospect of a direct benefit both to the pregnant woman and the fetus, or no prospect of benefit for the woman nor the fetus when risk to the fetus is not greater than minimal and the purpose of the research is the development of important biomedical knowledge that cannot be obtained by any other means, her consent is obtained in accord with the informed consent provisions of subpart A of this part;

(e) If the research holds out the prospect of direct benefit solely to the fetus then the consent of the pregnant woman and the father is obtained in accord with the informed consent provisions of subpart A of this part, except that the father's consent need not be obtained if he is unable to consent because of unavailability, incompetence, or temporary incapacity or the pregnancy resulted from rape or incest.

(f) Each individual providing consent under paragraph (d) or (e) of this section is fully informed regarding the reasonably foreseeable impact of the research on the fetus or neonate;

(g) For children as defined in § 46.402(a) who are pregnant, assent and permission are obtained in accord with the provisions of subpart D of this part."[11]

are based, that can be corroborated by accepted scientific methods of observation and inference. In the present context, 'research' includes both medical and behavioral studies pertaining to human health."[10] In the United States, human subjects research is regulated by the federal government under Title 45 Part 46 of the Code of Federal Regulations (45 CFR 46), *Protection of Human Subjects*, known as the Common Rule. It defines research as follows: "*Research* means a systematic investigation, including research development, testing and evaluation, designed to develop or contribute to generalizable knowledge."[11] Both of these definitions agree that the purpose of clinical research, both retrospective and prospective, is primarily to benefit future patients by producing generalizable knowledge. This is not to say that clinical research never clinically benefits an individual subject, but it is to say that this is not its *primary* purpose.

The Common Rule provides guidance specific to perinatal research for maternal or fetal benefit. (The pertinent text of this section appears in Table 8.1) Subsection (a) calls for a foundation for proposed research in prior research and for conducting such research, if it has not been already completed, when "scientifically appropriate." Ezekiel Emanuel et al. provide a helpful compilation of seven ethical requirements of ethical research that can be found in twentieth-century sources, including scientific value and validity,[10] the focus of Subsection (a). The importance of a solid scientific foundation for clinical research was recognized as early in the history of research ethics as the eighteenth century by Dr. John Gregory (1724–1773) of Scotland, who wrote the first modern medical ethics in the English language.[12] He developed a research ethics to address the potential abuse of patients in the Royal Infirmary of Edinburgh by younger physicians anxious to establish their reputations. These physicians would pronounce Infirmary patients incurable, not to abandon them (which was then the common practice), but to justify introducing experimental medicines of their own invention.

Gregory condemned this practice. His first justification was that such experimentation was clinically premature: standard remedies had not yet been attempted and shown to be ineffective in a patient's care. His second justification was that experimentation was often poorly designed. For example, compound drugs would be used without attention to the question of which elements of the compound might cause observed clinical effects. His third justification was that such physicians used the sick poor to advance their own reputational interests, subjecting them to unnecessary risk of clinical harm out of personal self-interest. Gregory was concerned to prevent "sporting" with the sick poor, what we now call exploitation, a justice-based concept introduced in Chapter 3: using others to advance one's own interests or the interest of a small group, oblivious to the harm such use may cause to many others who will not experience the opportunity for an offsetting benefit.

We invoke Gregory's research ethics because it has important, but insufficiently appreciated implications for how to interpret the requirement of establishing the scientific value and validity of research in pregnant women or fetuses. From this eighteenth-century perspective, Subsection (a) should be interpreted to mean that such research should be undertaken only when standard remedies have been attempted and reliably judged to be futile, i.e. reliably expected not to achieve their outcomes for protecting the health or life of the pregnant woman or fetus. Such research should also be well designed. This now means that there should be a focused research question and hypotheses, the testing of which is reliably expected to answer the research question. For clinically unprecedented research on pregnant women or fetuses, this means that there must at least be animal studies or simulations, the results of which are sufficient to refine the focused research question and explore the testability of its hypotheses. Investigators should not allow the drive for advancement, recognition, and increased market share – all sources of potential conflicts of interest in Gregory's day and certainly in ours – to bias the research design. Gregory emphasized that adherence to the intellectual and moral demands of scientific rigor provides the antidote to such bias, a view that originated in the philosophy of science of Francis Bacon (1561–1626), which Gregory cites and which is implicit in Subsection (a).

Emanuel et al.[10] identify the informed consent of human subjects of research as one of the ethical requirements that can be found in twentieth-century sources, such as the Nuremberg Code that was issued at the conclusion of the Nazi Medical War Crimes trials[13] and the Declaration of Helsinki.[14] Informed consent became a component of research ethics as early as the nineteenth century.[15] Subsection (d) calls for the informed consent of adult pregnant women, while Subsection (g) calls for assent of legal minors who are pregnant. Subsection (f) requires that the scope of information to be provided includes risks to the fetus or neonate. Subsection (e) requires consent of the father of the fetus for research designed to benefit the fetus. While this is an ethically controversial requirement, it must be satisfied for research conducted under an IRB-approved protocol in the U. S.

Subsections (b) and (c) concern what Emanuel et al. call the ethical requirement of a favorable risk-benefit ratio.[10] This requires the minimization of risk to the life and health of research subjects, the "enhancement of potential benefits," and proportionality of the risks to the expected health benefits to future patients and society. Subsection (b) distinguishes research that is designed to have "the prospect of direct benefit for the woman or fetus" from research that does not and has the purpose of developing "important biomedical knowledge which cannot be obtained by any other means." Subsection (c) requires minimization of risk "for achieving the objectives of the research." For research without the prospect of direct benefit to the woman or fetus, Subsection (b) requires that the risk to the fetus is "not greater than minimal." Section 46.102(i) defines minimal risk as follows: "*Minimal risk* means that the probability and magnitude of harm or discomfort anticipated in the research are not greater in and of themselves than those ordinarily encountered in daily life or during the performance of routine physical or psychological examinations or tests."[11] The concept of minimal risk does *not* apply to research that does have the prospect of direct benefit to the pregnant woman or fetus, the focus of this chapter. No guidance is provided on how to assess risk to the fetus of research that is designed to directly benefit pregnant women or fetuses.

8.4 The central ethical challenge

The central ethical challenge in research with the prospect of direct benefit to the pregnant woman or fetus is to provide such guidance, i.e. a framework for making ethically justified judgments about the nature and severity of risks to the pregnant woman and fetus in order to reliably determine that the risk-benefit ratio is indeed favorable. Emanuel et al. state that the justifying ethical values for a favorable risk-benefit ratio are "[n]on-maleficence, beneficence, and non-exploitation,"[10] with the latter being a justice-based concern. As pointed out above, Gregory already insisted on non-exploitation as a core component of research ethics. The ethical principles of beneficence and nonmaleficence are certainly well known in contemporary bioethics.[16,17] (See Chapter 1) Both, of course, have deep roots in the history of Western medical ethics, although the first use of 'beneficence' as we use it – the ethical principle that obligates the physician to seek the greater balance of clinical goods over clinical harms in patient care – is probably in Thomas Percival's (1740–1804) *Medical Ethics*, the first book with that title in any language in the global history of medical ethics.[18]

To explain the minimization of risk, Emanuel et al. quote without further elaboration Section 46.111(a)(1) on the minimization of risk: "Risks to subjects are minimized: (i) By using procedures which are consistent with sound research design and which do not unnecessarily expose subjects to risk, and (ii) whenever appropriate, by using procedures already being performed on the subjects for diagnostic or treatment purposes."[10,11] They go on to state that "potential benefits to individual subjects from the research are delineated and enhanced."[11] They insist that only "health-related benefits" be included. Assessment of the risk-benefit ratio "can appeal to explicit standards, informed by existing data on the potential types of harms and benefits, their likelihood of occurring, and their long-term consequences,"[10] referencing the Belmont Report of the U. S. National Commission for the Protection of Human Subjects.[19] On this approach to research ethics, judgments about risk, benefit, and the risk-benefit ratio are *clinical* judgments about health-related benefits and risks, i.e. judgments about the application of the ethical principles of nonmaleficence, beneficence, and justice to subjects as if they were *patients*. Implicit in this approach to assessing the risk-benefit ratio is the view that clinical investigators have a fiduciary responsibility to protect research subjects from unacceptable harm, i.e. *net* clinical harm, which would violate the ethical principles of nonmaleficence and beneficence.

Deliberative clinical ethical judgment about an acceptable risk-benefit ratio for the pregnant woman, in research designed to benefit pregnant women as well as in research designed to benefit the fetus, comes under the purview of perinatal ethics. Such clinical ethical judgment will be complex in both kinds of clinical research but its basis is clear.

It is less clear what the basis of clinical ethical judgment about a favorable risk-benefit ratio for the fetus should be. Section 46.204 provides no guidance as to the basis for assessing risk to the fetus and requires only that it be minimized. Baruch Brody has pointed out, correctly, that the earlier version of the Common Rule "is really quite permissive. When the research is therapeutic research (the purpose being to "meet the health needs of the mother"), there is no requirement that maternal and fetal interests be balanced. The only requirement is that the fetus not be placed at more risk than is necessary to meet the maternal health need."[4] This analysis pertains to Section 46.204 as well. Clinical risk to the fetus is to be minimized by selecting the least risky research design that is adequate to test the hypotheses. Whether such relative clinical risk is intrinsically acceptable depends on assessment of the risk in terms of "the potential types of harms and benefits, their likelihood of occurring, and their long-term consequences."[10] In other words, Emanuel, Wendler, and Grady's analysis is meant to be clinical.

Deliberative clinical ethical judgment about an acceptable risk-benefit ratio for the fetus, in research designed to benefit pregnant women as well as in research designed to benefit the fetus, comes under the purview of obstetric ethics. A core component of obstetric ethics is the ethical concept of the fetus as a patient, as explained in Chapter 1. The ethical concept of the fetus as a patient is, therefore, essential to applying the ethical requirement of a favorable risk-benefit ratio to the fetus for research intended to benefit either the pregnant woman or the fetus.

8.5 Research designed to improve the health of pregnant women

Lylerly et al. call attention to the wide range of research that needs to be undertaken to improve the health of pregnant women.[3] They include the clinical management of hypertension and diabetes, psychiatric disorders and illnesses such as depression, cancer, and polypharmacy.

We have argued for clinical ethical criteria for pharmacologic research on pregnant women that is designed to improve their health[20] and we have applied these criteria to the ethics of placebo-controlled clinical trials of antidepressants in pregnant women.[21] Here, we generalize these criteria to address both medical and surgical research intended to benefit the pregnant woman and to address innovation as well as Phases I, II, and III clinical investigation. We present criteria for the initiation of innovation and Phase I and Phase II clinical trials (Table 8.2) and then for the initiation of randomized controlled clinical trials (Table 8.3).

The first criterion in Tables 8.2 and 8.3 should guide judgments about the scientific value of proposed research and the application of Section 46.204(a). These criteria reflect Gregory's prescient concern to prevent scientifically premature research, by emphasizing the need for an evidence base for a reasonable expectation of improvement of pregnant women's health from preceding animal

Table 8.2: Ethical criteria for innovation and initiation phase I and II clinical trials to improve the health of pregnant patients.

1. The medical or surgical intervention should be reliably expected to be efficacious in managing the pregnant woman's diagnosis: there is a reasonable expectation of prevention of serious, far-reaching, and irreversible clinical sequelae of her diagnosis. The evidence-base for this clinical judgment should include all previous animal and human studies. Medications or surgeries with an evidence-base that supports reasonable expectation of efficacy should receive priority for preliminary investigation with pregnant women. Medications or surgeries without such an evidence-base should not receive priority for clinical investigation.
2. There should be no documented mortality or documented serious, far-reaching, and irreversible injury to the fetal patient, especially to the central nervous system, sensory system, or other major organ system from use of the medication or performance of the surgery.
3. There should be no or very low documented risk of less serious injury to the fetal patient.

Table 8.3: Ethical criteria for initiating randomized controlled clinical trials to improve the health of pregnant patients.

1. In preliminary studies, such as Phase 1 and 2 or cohort studies, the medication or surgery has demonstrated efficacy in preventing serious, far-reaching, and irreversible clinical sequelae of the pregnant woman's diagnosis.
2. In these preliminary studies, there have been no documented cases, attributable to the investigational drug or surgery, of mortality or of serious, far-reaching, and irreversible injury to the fetal patient, especially to the central nervous system, sensory system, or other major organ system.
3. There should be no or only rare documented occurrences of less serious injury to the fetal patient.

and human investigation. This criterion is also designed to discipline innovation of new interventions and also to reduce the bias that reputational and other forms of self-interest can introduce into such exciting areas of clinical research.

The ethical concept of the fetus as a patient shapes the second and third criteria for Phase I and Phase II research (Table 8.2) and for Phase III research (Table 8.3), which concern judgments about the risk-benefit ratio and provide the guidance that is lacking in Section 46.204 for its Subsections (b) and (c). These criteria employ different ethical strategies to prevent exploitation of both the pregnant and fetal patients. The fetal patient is vulnerable in the sense that it is incapable of consenting to involvement in research to benefit the pregnant woman. The investigator, therefore, has a professional, justice-based to protect such a patient from exploitation, i.e. being subjected to serious clinical harm with no opportunity to experience offsetting clinical benefit. To prevent exploitation of the pregnant woman, these criteria define causally stringent parameters of mortality and morbidity as the basis for judgments about whether a specific research design has acceptable risks to the fetal patient and has, therefore, minimized them. In particular, fetal mortality is included as an unacceptable outcome, because the fetus cannot consent to this risk. These two criteria also satisfy the requirement of Section 46.204(c) to minimize risk to the fetus, by stringently defining the boundaries of intrinsically acceptable risk. We emphasize that these criteria concern minimized risk, not minimal risk, which conceptually does not apply to assessing the risk-benefit ratio in research to benefit the pregnant woman.

8.6 Research designed to improve medical and surgical management of the fetal patient

The need for an ethical framework for innovators and PIRCS and for investigators and IRBs/RECs is not limited to the ethics of research to benefit the pregnant woman. The burgeoning area of fetal medicine and surgery means that investiga-

Table 8.4: Ethical criteria for innovation and initiation phase I and II clinical trials to improve the health of fetal patients.

1. The proposed fetal intervention is reliably expected on the basis of previous animal studies either to be life-saving or to prevent serious and irreversible disease, injury, or disability for the fetal patient;
2. Among possible alternative designs, the intervention is designed in such a way as to involve the least risk of mortality and morbidity to the fetal patient; and
3. On the basis of animal studies and analysis of theoretical risks both for the current and future pregnancies, the mortality risk to the pregnant woman is reliably expected to be low and the risk of disease, injury, or disability to the pregnant woman is reliably expected to be low or manageable for current and future pregnancies.

Table 8.5: Ethical criteria for evidence-based equipoise and therefore for initiating randomized controlled clinical trials to improve the health of fetal patients.

1. The initial case series indicates that the proposed fetal intervention is reliably expected either to be life saving or to prevent serious and irreversible disease, injury, or disability for the fetal patient;
2. Among possible alternative designs, the intervention continues to involve the least risk of morbidity and mortality to the fetal patient; and
3. The case series indicates that the mortality risk to the pregnant woman is reliably expected to be low and the risk of disease, injury, or disability to the pregnant woman, including for future pregnancies, is reliably expected to be low or manageable.

tors and IRBs/RECs will also need an ethical framework for research to improve the medical and surgical management of the fetal patient.[6]

We have argued for clinical ethical criteria for surgical research on pregnant women that is designed to improve the health of fetal patients.[5] Here, we generalize these criteria to address medical and surgical interventions for fetal benefit and to address innovation as well as Phases I, II, and III clinical investigation. We present criteria for the initiation of innovation and Phase I and Phase II clinical trials (Table 8.4) and then for the initiation of randomized controlled clinical trials (Table 8.5).

The first criterion in Tables 8.4 and 8.5 should guide judgments about the scientific value of proposed research and the application of Section 46.204(a). These criteria also reflect Gregory's prescient concern to prevent scientifically premature research. This criterion is also designed to discipline innovation of new interventions for fetal benefit and also to reduce the bias that reputational and other forms of self-interest can introduce into such exciting areas of clinical research.

The ethical concept of the fetus as a patient shapes the second and third criteria for Phase I and Phase II research (Table 8.4) and for Phase III research (Table 8.5), which concern judgments about the risk-benefit ratio and provide the guidance that is lacking in Section 46.204 for its Subsections (b) and (c). These two criteria employ different ethical strategies to prevent exploitation of both the pregnant and fetal patients.

These criteria invoke the ethical concept of the fetus as a patient and the physician's professional, beneficence-based responsibility to protect patients not capable of consent to exposure to risk of harm and to balance beneficence-based obligations to the fetal patient with beneficence-based and autonomy based obligations to the pregnant woman. The second criterion in Tables 3 and 4 makes explicit the beneficence-based obligation to protect the health and life of the fetal patient. Criterion 2, on the minimization of risk, we emphasize, does not prohibit risk of mortality to the fetal patient, as the concept of minimal risk might. This criterion does require that this risk be minimized by the selection of study design with the lowest predicted risk of mortality. As required by the professional responsibility model of perinatal ethics, the third criterion in Tables 8.4 and 8.5 takes into account both the beneficence-based obligation to protect the health and life of the pregnant woman and the autonomy-based obligation to respect her decision about how much risk she is willing to take for herself. Both criteria are required by the ethical concept of the fetus as a patient. Unlike the fetal patient, the pregnant woman can consent, and it is not ethically unacceptable to use medication or perform surgery that involves an acceptably low (in beneficence-based clinical judgment) risk of mortality for a non-pregnant patient, provided that the patient is informed about and consents to this risk. The ethical criteria for research to benefit the fetus in Tables 8.4 and 8.5 reflect this major ethical difference between pregnant patients and fetal patients. The pregnant woman is in a position to protect herself from potential exploitation for the potential benefit of the fetal patient because she has no beneficence-based obligation to the fetal patient to enroll in a clinical trial. Her refusal to do so, therefore, violates no beneficence-based obligations to the fetal patient. These matters must be made clear in the informed consent process.

The results of Phase I and II research should be carefully evaluated, using the criteria for initiating Phase III research. When these criteria are satisfied, one of the necessary conditions for Phase III research, the existence of evidence-based equipoise, is satisfied. Evidence-based equipoise means that deliberative clinical judgment about the outcomes of Phase I and II studies requires the judger to become uncertain whether the new form of medical or surgical intervention is clinically superior to current medical or surgical management. Evidence-based equipoise should be distinguished from opinion-equipoise, an empirical observation that the relevantly experienced research community is roughly equally divided about whether the new form of medical or surgical intervention is clinically superior to current medical or surgical management.

An ethics of fetal research based on concepts and discourses of personhood, fetal rights, or the unborn child, would treat the fetal patient as a separate patient, and therefore not necessarily take account of beneficence-based obligations to pregnant women. An ethics of research that rejected personhood, fetal rights, and the unborn child would not necessarily take account of beneficence-based obligations to the fetal patient. The third criterion in Tables 8.4 and 8.5 makes explicit the beneficence-based obligation to protect the pregnant woman's future pregnancies, not just her current pregnancy.

Some have proposed that fetal surgery and, by extension, fetal research, be designated as maternal-fetal surgery or research.[22] The ethical concept of the fetus as a patient supports this nomenclature only when it requires that beneficence-based obligations to the fetal patient and autonomy-based and beneficence-based obligations to the pregnant *all* be taken into account. The ethical concept of the fetus as a patient does *not* support this nomenclature if it excludes or systematically subordinates to the pregnant patient beneficence-based obligations owed to the fetal patient, i.e. especially if this discourse masks an appeal to the maternal-rights reductionist approach to perinatal ethics (see Chapter 1).

8.7 Responsibly managing the transition from investigation to clinical practice

The purpose of clinical investigation is to determine whether there is a reliable evidence-base for transitioning an investigational intervention into clinical practice. In other words, has the investigation shown that the intervention should now no longer be regarded as investigational but as medically reasonable alternative, i.e. clinical management for which there is an evidence base of net clinical benefit, that should be offered in the future for the clinical management of a maternal or fetal diagnosis?

We have argued for such criteria,[5] and here we generalize them to address both medical and surgical research and both maternal and fetal research (Table 8.6). These criteria are designed to responsibly manage the transition from investigation to clinical practice under the synergistic discipline of both evidence-based reasoning and argument-based ethical reasoning (see Chapter 10). These criteria reflect the complexity of clinical ethical judgment required by the ethical concept

Table 8.6: Ethical criteria for responsibly managing the transition from investigation to clinical practice.

1. The maternal or fetal intervention has positive results, i.e. it has a significant probability of being life-saving or preventing serious or irreversible disease, injury, or disability for the pregnant woman or fetal patient.
2. The maternal or fetal intervention involves low mortality and low or manageable risk of serious and irreversible disease, injury, or disability to the fetal patient, and
3. The mortality risk to the pregnant woman is low and the risk of disease, injury or disability is low or manageable, including for future pregnancies.

of the fetus as a patient. For maternal research, the ethical concept of the fetus as a patient justifies the second criterion, which makes explicit beneficence-based obligations to protect the life and health of the fetal patient. For fetal research, the ethical concept of the fetus as a patient justifies both the second criterion and the third criterion, which expresses beneficence-based obligations to the pregnant woman. The third criterion in Tables 8.6 makes explicit the beneficence-based obligation to protect the pregnant woman's future pregnancies, not just the current pregnancy.

8.8 Conclusion

The professional responsibility model of perinatal ethics calls for the improvement of perinatal practice by initiating a disciplined pathway from innovation as pre-research with PIRC approval into early-phase research with IRB/REC approval or by initiating early phase research with IRB/REC approval. The result of early-phase research should be carefully evaluated, to reach a deliberative clinical ethical judgment that Phase III research is warranted because in evidence-based equipoise exists. The results of all phases of research should be carefully evaluated in reaching a deliberative clinical ethical judgment so that the transition from research into clinical practice is scientifically, clinically, and ethically justified.

The core ethical consideration throughout the process of designing, conducting, and evaluating perinatal research is the assessment of the risk-benefit ratio for both the pregnant woman and fetus from a clinical perspective. The professional responsibility model of perinatal ethics and its ethical concept of the fetus as a patient play essential roles in creating such a framework and insulating it from the divisive and intractable abortion debate. Keeping that debate out of the ethics of research on pregnant women allows protocols to be developed and assessed on their scientific and ethical merits, not on their political acceptability to whichever faction of the debate holds power at any particular time. The comprehensive set of ethically justified criteria, provide the needed guidance. The professional responsibility model also guides the transition from research to clinical practice. As professionally responsible perinatal innovation and research advance, appropriate ethical guidance will facilitate improvement of the health of pregnant women and fetal patients in a scientifically disciplined and morally responsible fashion.

8.9 References

1. Chervenak FA, McCullough LB. An ethically justified framework for clinical investigation to benefit pregnant and fetal patients. Am J Bioeth 2011;11:39–49.
2. Chervenak FA, McCullough LB. Scientifically and ethically responsible innovation and research in ultrasound in obstetrics and gynecology. Ultrasound Obstet Gynecol 2006;28:1–4.

3. Lyerly AD, Little MO, Faden RR. 2008. Pregnancy and clinical research. Hastings Cent Rept 2008;38:53.
4. Brody BA. 1998. The Ethics of Biomedical Research: An International Perspective. New York: Oxford University Press, 1998.
5. Chervenak FA, McCullough LB. 2002. A comprehensive ethical framework for fetal research and its application to fetal surgery for spina bifida. Am J Obstet Gynecol 2002;187:10–14.
6. Harrison MA, Evans MI, Adzick NS, Holzgreve W. 2001. The Unborn Patient: The Art and Science of Fetal Therapy, 3d. ed. Philadelphia: W.B. Saunders Company, 2001.
7. Biffl WL, Spain DA, Reitsma AM et al. Society of University Surgeons Surgical Innovations Project Team. Responsible development and application of surgical innovations: a position statement of the Society of University Surgeons. J Am Coll Surg 2008;206:1204–1209.
8. McNeally MF, Daar AS. Introducing new technologies: protecting subjects of surgical innovation and research. World J Surg 2003;27:930–935.
9. Reitsma AM, Moreno JD. Ethical regulations for innovative surgery: the last frontier? J Am Coll Surg, 2002;194:792–801.
10. Council of the International Organization of Medical Societies. International Ethical Guidelines for Biomedical Research Involving Human Subjects. 2002. www.cioms.ch/publications/guidelines/guidelines_nov_2002_blurb.htm, accessed March 2, 2014.
11. Department of Health and Human Services, "Protection of Human Subjects," 45 CFR 46. Available at www.hhs.gov/ohrp/humansubjects/guidance/45cfr46.html, accessed March 2, 2014.
12. McCullough LB. John Gregory and the Invention of Professional Medical Ethics and the Profession of Medicine. Dordrecht, The Netherlands: Kluwer Academic Publishers, 1998.
13. Schmidt U. Medical ethics and Nazism. In Vaker RB, McCullough LB, eds. The Cambridge World History of Medical Ethics. New York: Cambridge University Press, 2009:595–608.
14. World Medical Association. Declaration of Helsinki – Ethical principles for medical research involving human subjects. 2013. Available at www.wma.net/en/30publications/10policies/b3/, accessed March 2, 2014.
15. Lederer SE. The ethics of experimenting on human subjects. In Baker RB, McCullough LB, eds., The Cambridge World History of Medical Ethics. New York: Cambridge University Press, 2009:558–565.
16. Beauchamp TL, Childress JF. Principles of Biomedical Ethics, 7th ed. New York: Oxford University Press, 2012.
17. McCullough LB, Chervenak, FA. Ethics in Obstetrics and Gynecology. New York: Oxford University Press, 1994.
18. Percival T. Medical Ethics, or a Code of Institutes and Precepts adapted to the Professional Conduct of Physicians and Surgeons. London: Printed by S. Russell for J. Johnson and R. Bickerstaff, 1803.
19. National Commission for the Protection of Human Subjects of Biomedical and Behavioral Research. The Belmont Report. Washington, DC: U. S. Government Printing Office, 1979.
20. McCullough LB, Coverdale JH, Chervenak, FA. A comprehensive ethical framework for responsibly designing and conducting pharmacologic research that involves pregnant women. Am J Obstet Gynecol 2005;193(Pt.2):901–907.
21. Coverdale JH, McCullough LB, Chervenak FA. The ethics of randomized placebo-controlled trials of antidepressants with pregnant women: a systematic review. Obstet Gynecol 2008;112:1361–1368.
22. Lyerly AD, Gates EA, Cefalo RC, Sugarman JS. Toward the ethical evaluation and use of maternal-fetal surgery. Obstet Gynecol 2001;98:689–697.

8.10 Summary points

- Innovation and research are both forms of experimentation, because their outcomes cannot be reliably predicted in deliberative clinical judgment.
- Innovation is an experiment undertaken to benefit a pregnant or fetal patient.
- Research is undertaken to produce generalizable knowledge that aims to improve the quality of perinatal care.
- Planned innovation should be prospectively reviewed and approved for its scientific, clinical, and ethical justification by a Perinatal Innovation Review Committee.
- When such innovation has promising results, its next use should be either in planned innovation prospectively reviewed and approved for its scientific, clinical, and ethical justification by a Perinatal Innovation Review Committee or in early-phase research prospectively reviewed and approved by an Institutional Review Board/Research Ethics Committee.
- Phase I, II, and III research, to benefit pregnant patients, should be prospectively reviewed and approved for its scientific, clinical, and ethical justification by an Institutional Review Board/Research Ethics Committee.
- Phase I, II, and III, to benefit fetal patients, should be prospectively reviewed and approved for its scientific, clinical, and ethical justification by an Institutional Review Board/Research Ethics Committee.
- The transition from planned innovation and research to clinical practice should be responsibly managed on the basis of deliberative clinical ethical judgment.

9 Women and children first: Advocacy in perinatal medicine

9.1 Introduction

The professional responsibility model of perinatal ethics applies not only to clinical practice and research, but also to the perinatologist's role as advocate for the effective prevention and clinical management of the conditions, diseases, disorders, and injuries of pregnant, fetal, and neonatal patients.[1] This chapter provides ethical guidance for doing so, on the basis of the traditional invocation of "Women and children first."

9.2 "Women and children first"

"Women and children first" is certainly a familiar phrase but its origin is less well known. In 1852 the HMS Birkenhead, with more than 600 sailors, troops, and civilians aboard, was evacuating the civilians from Cape Town, South Africa during the Cape Frontier War (1850–1853). At 2 am on the morning of February 26, she struck unchartered rocks near Danger Point and began to take on water and then to sink. The number of lifeboats was not sufficient to convey all safely off the doomed ship. Many of the troops on board drowned in their berths as the ship foundered. The remaining men and officers of the 74th Regiment of Foot were mustered on deck by their commanding officer, Lt. Colonel Seton. He realized the nature of the situation and ordered his men to stand fast while the women and children were boarded onto the lifeboats. His soldiers obeyed and went down with the ship.[3] While it is not known whether Lt. Colonel Seton used the phrase, "women and children first," he is credited with being among the first to put it into practice. His heroism and that of his men allowed the women and children on board to be saved.

The Birkenhead incident occurred during a period of British imperialism and colonialism. Any incident from such a time would seem to be out of place as an exemplar for medical ethics and health policy today. We think otherwise: making "women and children first" was a defining moment in the history of world civilizations, and therefore has direct relevance for healthcare today.

The sad reality is that women and children are not first in our world; indeed, they are often last. This is especially the case in developing countries, which often do not provide adequate health care for women and children, as reflected perinatal mortality rates.[4] International organizations, such as UNICEF,[4] the World Health Organization,[5] and the World Bank,[6] and international associations of physicians, such as FIGO,[7] Matres Mundi,[8] and the World Association of Perinatal Medicine,[9] have led major efforts to identify problems in obstetric and neonatal care in developing countries and have advocated for improvement. The International Academy of Perinatal Medicine has added its voice to these advocacy efforts, with its "New York Declaration" on "Woman and Children First," which was presented at the United Nations on July 7, 2008, by. The Declaration defined sources of bias against the just allocation of healthcare resources for women and children in the developing world.[1]

The lack of prioritization for healthcare for women and children is not confined to developing countries. This can also be a problem in the United States and other developed countries. This chapter deploys the professional responsibility model of perinatal medicine to provide perinatologists with effective tools to advocate for the just allocation of healthcare resources for women and children. This is an especially timely topic for American obstetricians, where the Affordable Care Act of 2011, known informally as Obamacare, should increase the resources available to care for pregnant, fetal, and neonatal patients. Perinatologists can and should advocate for the priority of women and children in a world that had been largely dominated by politics and, at times, by injustice.

9.3 Justice-based professional responsibility

Advocacy for the healthcare needs of pregnant, fetal, and neonatal patients appeals to the ethical principle of justice, because it addresses the fair allocation of healthcare resources, a key component of professional responsibility.[10,11] In general, the ethical principle of justice requires that we render to each individual and to organizations what is due to them, a concept of justice that originates in the philosophy of Aristotle.[11] The crucial word in this formulation is "due." What is due to each individual or organization is fair treatment, which can be understood in two related ways.

The first sense of justice as fairness concerns the outcome of the decision making process. This is known as substantive justice.[10] Substantive justice requires that the reasons for setting priorities among competing interests of stakeholders, which determine the outcome of the decision-making process, be persuasive. There are competing accounts in ethical theory about which reasons should count as persuasive, and therefore about which actual allocations of scarce resources are fair. In the course of our analysis of challenges to substantive justice in the allocation of healthcare for women and children in healthcare policy, we will identify and justify the reasons that should be invoked to guide responses to these challenges.

The second sense of justice as fairness concerns a fair process or procedure for allocating scarce resources. This is known as procedural justice.[10] Procedural justice requires that interests of every individual and organization affected by the allocation of scarce resources should have his, her, or its interests identified and taken into account in the decision-making process. In the course of our analysis of challenges to procedural justice in the allocation of healthcare for women and children in healthcare policy, we will identify how the interests of pregnant, fetal, and neonatal patients should be taken into account as the basis for responding to these challenges.

9.4 Challenges to justice in the allocation of healthcare resources to women and children

Challenges to justice in the allocation of healthcare resources to women and children in the United States arise for both substantive and procedural justice. We address each set of challenges in turn.

9.4.1 Challenges to substantive justice

Challenges to substantive justice include the self-interest of adults, age bias, and economic bias. There can be two kinds of economic bias: against pregnant, fetal, and neonatal patients; and against obstetric services.

Self-interest of adults. The first challenge to substantive justice in the allocation of healthcare resources to women and children arises from self-interest. Adults will never again be fetal or neonatal patients, but virtually all will be patients at some time(s) in their lives, especially as they age and, for many, also experience chronic disease and disability. In a society with a lower replacement birth rate among some subpopulations than in the past, such as the United States, the self-interest of adults who have not or will not have children may be another source of self-interest in having healthcare resources allocated to themselves. These sources of self-interest create a major challenge to substantive justice in the allocation of healthcare resources to women and children.

The response to this challenge draws on the professional responsibility of perinatologists to fulfill their beneficence-based obligation to protect and promote the health-related interests of patients (see Chapter 1). By its very nature, professional responsibility to patients is not a function of the patient's age or interest in having children. It follows that, for physicians, the healthcare interests of one population of patients should not be neglected in order to advance the healthcare interests of another population of patients. Allocating healthcare resources based on the self-interest of one population of patients, when doing so results in inadequate resources for another population of patients, is not compatible with the professional responsibility model of perinatal ethics. Physicians should, therefore, identify and expose such inadequate allocations of healthcare resources as violations of substantive justice based on professional ethical considerations.

Age bias. A closely related challenge is age bias. In the United States, public funding of healthcare favors the elderly, in the form of Medicare, which enjoys broad and enduring political support. In 1965, when Medicare was enacted, millions of elderly Americans risked being plunged into poverty or near-poverty by major illness requiring hospitalization. President Johnson argued that this was not acceptable, because of the sacrifices that the older generation had made, especially during the Great Depression, and that aging cohorts had made in World War II. This was sound ethical reasoning, because it appealed to reciprocal justice: those who have sacrificed for society's good have a legitimate claim on society's resources. The commitment to prevent medically induced poverty among the elderly remains sound ethical reasoning.

The response to this ethical challenge is not to argue against Medicare and other public support for the elderly, because substantive justice does not support such a response. Instead, obstetricians should invoke the life-cycle principle to argue for increased priority for healthcare resources for children.[12] This ethical principle holds that everyone should have an opportunity to live and develop through all stages of life. The younger one is, the more years one is expected to live. This creates a priority for allocating healthcare resources to the youngest, fetal and neonatal patients, and, by necessity, pregnant women. The resources that fulfilling such a priority requires, while substantial, are not of the scale as Medicare. Allocating healthcare resources to women and children may be cost-saving, e.g. from improved outcomes of pregnancy. In addition, healthier children are more likely to become productive members of society and repay the investment in their healthcare many times over economically, socially, and other important ways.

A second variant of substantive justice is also relevant, i.e. the investment refinement principle, which has direct implications for substantive justice in the allocation of healthcare resources to pregnant women. This ethical principle "emphasizes gradations within a life span. It gives priority to people between early adolescence and middle age on the basis of the amount the person invested in his or her life balanced by the amount left to live."[12] Pregnant women are in this category and have an enormous biopsychosocial investment in pregnancies being taken to term and the lives of their future children. With good obstetric (and other medical) care, pregnant women can be expected to live for many years and their children even longer. The investment refinement principle is therefore abundantly satisfied and creates a powerful response to the challenge of age bias by justifying allocation of healthcare resources to pregnant women.

Economic bias against pregnant, fetal, and neonatal patients. We believe that there is a general bias against the medically indigent in the United States. Medicare's justification was and remains reciprocal justice: to those who have sacrificed much for others and society, much is owed. It can be argued that poverty or near-poverty resulting from major illness is not the fault of the elderly and so such poverty is undeserved. In an older discourse from eighteenth-century Britain, which came to the North American British colonies, the elderly poor were considered the worthy poor. This contrasts with the eighteenth-century concept of the unworthy poor, those who are able but unwilling to work and support themselves, and therefore have no justice-based of reciprocity on society.[13]

The phrases "worthy poor" and "unworthy poor" are no longer in use, but the concepts may continue to shape healthcare policy in the United States. Medicaid, a state-federal program of healthcare for the medically indigent, is not adequately funded, unlike Medicare. Medicaid also has much lower reimbursement schedules than Medicare. The precarious funding of Medicaid, compared to Medicare, may reflect the historical and disturbing distinction between the unworthy and worthy poor, a form of economic bias.

This bias becomes especially vicious, and therefore egregiously unacceptable when it is applied to children of poverty and fetuses being carried by pregnant women of poverty. This is because impoverished fetal and neonatal patients and many impoverished pregnant women are not able to work and support themselves and are, therefore, not responsible for their poverty.

A powerful response to economic bias comes from the application of the ethical theory of justice of John Rawls (1921–2002), arguably the most important American political philosopher of the last century. Rawls' concern was that allocation of resources can seriously disadvantage the economically vulnerable, the "least well off" in his nomenclature. A utilitarian public policy would allocate resources to maximize the benefits to greatest number, but this could leave the situation of the least well off unchanged or even worse. Rawls sought to modify utilitarian substantive justice by arguing that such policy is ethically permissible only if it also improves the economic and social circumstances of the least well off. He called this the "maximin" principle.[14] Failure to constrain the utilitarian impulse by the maximin principle violates justice because unconstrained utilitarianism perpetuates exploitation, i.e. a situation in which some are benefited and many others are burdened with no or very limited opportunity to experience offsetting benefit.

The least well off, as we suggested above, can be understood in terms of vulnerability, the diminished ability to protect oneself. Fetal and neonatal patients are certainly among the most vulnerable patients, as are pregnant women who are impoverished. The substantive justice-based maximin principle is therefore justifiably invoked to make allocation of resources to fetal, neonatal, and impoverished pregnant patient a healthcare priority.

Economic bias against obstetric services. Unlike neonatal services, which are usually profit centers, there can also be economic bias against obstetric services in healthcare organizations, especially when they are considered distinctly. This bias results from what can be called the "trumping power" of economic values, which is distinct from economic bias against the poor. By "trumping power", we mean the tendency in public policy, and therefore in healthcare organizations, for economic concerns to override or even eliminate all other ethical considerations. This trumping becomes more pronounced when economies experience stagnant growth or contraction.

It is certainly a legitimate interest of healthcare organizations to be fiscally sound. To protect this legitimate interest, it is ethically permissible for healthcare organizations to emphasize higher margin clinical services, such as cardiovascular surgery, orthopedics, or oncology, and the profits they generate from high quality patient care. Ethical concern arises when other clinical services that may not be profitable may be cut back or eliminated, such as inpatient pediatrics. As a consequence, some patient populations come to be viewed as less valuable, and therefore less important than other patient populations, an organizational attitude that threatens professional integrity.[15]

The cost of professional liability insurance has hit obstetrics especially hard in many parts of the United States.[16] As a consequence, obstetrics' cost-profile can be markedly different from that of other specialties. The high cost of professional liability insurance for obstetrics in many states means that economic values gain trumping power at the level of healthcare organization leadership. The result is that obstetrics often comes to be seen exclusively as a cost center. This means that obstetrics can be viewed as a problem rather than a mission-vital clinical service. This can be manifest by a low prioritization for obstetrics in organizational philanthropic endeavors.

The response of perinatologists should be based on professional responsibility: no group of patients, grouped by specialties and their economic value to healthcare organizations, should count for less than any other group of patients. All groups of patients are important in professional medical ethics, whether or not one group of patients happens to generate more net revenues than another. Before making the case for organizational resources based on the equal importance of pregnant, fetal, and neonatal patients, leaders in obstetrics to get their financial houses in order, i.e. run obstetrics on a sound business basis.[17] Otherwise, legitimate advocacy will be subjected to unnecessary vulnerability.

There is tendency in all healthcare systems for economic values to trump or automatically override all other considerations, especially including professional integrity. As the great American folk singer and philosopher, Bob Dylan, once put it, "While money doesn't talk; it swears."[18] By getting their own financial houses in order, and advocating for the equal importance of pregnant, fetal, and neonatal patients, obstetricians will be in a position to talk back, countering the trumping power of economic considerations with advocacy for obstetric services as mission vital.

9.4.2 Challenges to procedural justice

There are also challenges to procedural justice. The first is bias in favor of persons, and the second is bias against those who cannot speak for themselves.

Bias in favor of persons. Persons in the ethics literature are understood to be human beings with independent moral status and autonomy. Personhood comes into existence only after birth and, on some accounts, not until the acquisition of language and social identity some time after birth. Personhood is a self-generated moral status, usually expressed in the language of rights.[19] The interests of stakeholders with personhood-based rights obviously have to be taken into account in order to meet the requirements of procedural justice.

Any claim that fetuses are also persons, and therefore have rights, is highly controversial in both philosophical ethics and theological ethics. As a consequence, fetuses are put at a competitive disadvantage in decision-making processes about allocation of resources, because their very status as stakeholders is in doubt, especially for those who think that only persons can be stakeholders. The result is a bias in procedural justice in favor of persons, because it assumes that only the interests of persons need to be taken into account.

Professional medical ethics provides a powerful antidote: the generation of interests from a human being's status as a patient, rather than a person. All patients have an interest in the protection and improvement of their health. Patients have this interest in virtue of being presented to a physician or other healthcare profession and the existence of clinical interventions that can protect and improve health. The genius of the ethical concept of the fetus as a patient is that it goes beyond the binomial of being a person or not, and therefore undercuts the biases generated by this categorization.

The way to take the interests of all patients into account is to recognize that all patients have an interest in being treated according to accepted standards of care. This applies to fetal patients, who are not yet persons, as well as to pregnant patients, who clearly are persons. Obstetricians should, therefore, point out that procedural justice requires that the interests of all patients be taken into account by those responsible for making and implementing healthcare policy. In particular, obstetricians should advocate that healthcare resources be made available to ensure that all patients are treated according to accepted standards of care.

Bias against those who cannot speak for themselves. Fetal and neonatal patients cannot speak for themselves in the policy-making process. In many cultures, pregnant women struggle to have their interests recognized and taken into account in setting healthcare priorities.[9] As a consequence, the health-related interests of fetal, neonatal, and pregnant patients may not be routinely taken into account on forming and implementing healthcare policy, which violates procedural justice.

Perinatologists are in a unique position to assume an advocacy role because they have expert scientific and clinical knowledge about how to identify and protect the health-related interests of fetal, neonatal, and pregnant patients.[9] On this basis, obstetricians should advocate for healthcare priorities that create resources to support the development and global implementation of evidence-based medical care for fetal, neonatal, and pregnant patients, so that their interests are taken into account in a scientific, unbiased fashion. The goal should be the elimination, to the greatest extent possible, of national and wide area variation in the processes and outcomes of obstetric care. Ideally, where a patient lives should not make a difference in the quality of medical care that the patient receives.

9.5 Conclusion

Perinatologists can become cynical about the ethical principle of justice because it appears abstract, and therefore to lack clinical application. This cynicism can be reinforced by their experience with the professional liability crisis.[16] The antidote to this understandable cynicism, and therefore to effective advocacy, is for perinatologists to renew their commitment to the professional responsibility model of perinatal ethics as it applies to the population of women and children. At this level, the model generates justice-based obligations to work for the resources required in deliberative clinical judgment to meet the healthcare needs of women and children. To fulfill these obligations, perinatologists should distinguish substantive and procedural justice, explicitly identify biases that distort organizational culture and healthcare policy, and use relevant concepts of justice to advocate for fetal, neonatal, and pregnant patients whose healthcare otherwise is at risk of unacceptable compromise. By focusing on the interests of patients and keeping their own self-interest secondary, obstetricians can advocate for their patients from the moral high ground of making women and children first as matter of justice and professional integrity.

9.6 References

1. Chervenak FA, McCullough LB, International Academy of Perinatal Medicine. Women and children first – or last? The New York Declaration. Am J Obstet Gynecol 2009;2001;35.
2. Chervenak FA, McCullough LB. Women and children first: transforming an historic defining moment into a contemporary ethical imperative. Am J Obstet Gynecol 2009;201:335.e1–5.
3. Historic UK.Com. "Women and children first" – the silent heroes of the Birkenhead. Available at www.historic-uk.com/CultureUK/WomenandChildrenFirst.htm, accessed March 2, 2014.
4. United Nations. UNICEF. www.unicef.org/, accessed March 2, 2014.
5. World Health Organization. www.who.int/en/, accessed March 2, 2014.
6. The World Bank. www.worldbank.org/, accessed March 2, 2014.
7. International Federation of Gynecology and Obstetrics. www.figo.org/, accessed March 2, 2014.
8. Matres Mundi. www.matres-mundi.org/, accessed June 19, 2014.
9. World Association of Perinatal Medicine. www.wapm.info/, accessed June 19, 2014.
10. Beauchamp TL, Childress JF. Principles of Biomedical Ethics, 7th ed. New York: Oxford University Press, 2012.
11. Aristotle. Nichomachean Ethics. Translated with an introduction and notes by Martin Oswald. Indianapolis: Boos-Merrill Company, 1962.
12. Emanuel EJ, Wertheimer A. Who should get influenza vaccine when not all can? Science 2006;312:854–855.

13. McCullough LB. John Gregory and the Invention of Professional Medical Ethics and the Profession of Medicine. Dordrecht, The Netherlands: Kluwer Academic Publishers, 1998.
14. Rawls J. A Theory of Justice. Cambridge, MA: Belknap Press of Harvard University, 1971. Revised edition 1999.
15. Chervenak FA, McCullough LB. The diagnosis and management of progressive dysfunction of healthcare organizations. Obstet Gynecol 2005;105:882–887.
16. Chervenak FA, McCullough LB. Neglected ethical dimensions of the professional liability crisis. Am J Obstet Gynecol 2004;190:1198–1200.
17. Chervenak FA, McCullough LB. Professionalism and justice: ethical management guidelines for leaders of academic medical centers. Acad Med 2002;77:45–47.
18. Bob Dylan. It's all right ma, I'm only bleeding. Lyrics available at www.bobdylan.com/#/songs/its-alright-ma-im-only-bleeding, accessed March 2, 2014.
19. McCullough LB, Chervenak FA. Ethics in Obstetrics and Gynecology. New York: Oxford University Press, 1994.

9.7 Summary points

- Perinatologists should identify and call public attention to biases that result in unjust allocations of healthcare resources for the care of pregnant, fetal, and neonatal patients.
- Perinatologists should advocate for the resources needed to address the healthcare needs of women and children as these are identified in deliberative clinical judgment, keeping self-interest systematically secondary.

10 Critically appraising the literature of perinatal ethics

10.1 Introduction

In Chapter 1, we described perinatal ethics as the disciplined study of the morality of perinatologists. As such, perinatal ethics seeks to identify the ethical obligations of perinatologists as these are generated by the professional responsibility model of perinatal ethics. The perinatal ethics literature, including the previous chapters in this book, offers ethical analyses and argument about the behavior and character of perinatologists that is required in an ethically appropriate practice of perinatology. Perinatologists will, we believe, benefit from having a tool that they can routinely use to critically appraise the literature of perinatal ethics.[1] In this chapter, we, therefore, set out a simple, four-step approach to appraising the perinatal ethics literature that is intentionally analogous to that taken in evidence-based medicine. We have adapted these four steps from those of evidence-based medicine, which are: (a) asking a focused question, (b) making a valid argument, (c) identifying the results of arguments, and (d) bringing the results of argument to clinical practice.[1]

10.2 Four-step approach

As we explained in Chapter 1, making ethical arguments is essential to well-reasoned perinatal ethics, and therefore to professional responsible perinatal practice, research, and advocacy. This is known as argument-based perinatal ethics or, more generally, argument-based ethics. Argument-based perinatal ethics should begin with a focused question that arises from actual experience in clinical practice. The purpose for asking a focused question is to produce argument-based conclusions that serve as valid and reliable answers to the question and thus as the basis for future decision making. Argument-based perinatal ethics should then undertake ethical analysis and argument, of which review of pertinent literature is a key component. The third step of argument-based perinatal ethics is to identify the conclusions of arguments clearly. The fourth step of argument-based perinatal ethics is to assess the applicability of these conclusions to the particular scenario that evoked the question in the first place, and to apply the results to the scenario when relevant.

10.2.1 Step 1: Does the argument address a focused ethics question?

To guide clinical judgment, decision making, and behavior in clinical practice, teaching, clinical research, and organizational culture, argument-based perinatal ethics begins with a clear, well-defined focus on a topic in clinical practice. There are a number of possible domains for a focused question, including theoretical issues (such as whether the fetus is a patient or a person), clinical issues for a specific patient population (the management of cancer during pregnancy), research issues for a specific population (surgical management of fetal spina bifida), organizational culture issues (quality improvement and cost control), and public policy issues (partial-birth abortion).

The ethical significance of the focused question should be explained. Its significance can be theoretical, as well as clinical. The perspective from which importance of the issue is claimed should be identified, including that of physicians, scientific investigators, patients, patient's families and other support networks, payers, health care organization leadership, and scholars and public officials concerned with health policy. The relevance of this consideration is that the target audience for the use of the results of the argument should be clear.

10.2.2 Step 2: Are the results of the argument valid?

The validity of the results in an ethics argument rests primarily on the quality of its ethical analysis and argument using clearly articulated concepts, as explained in Chapter 1. Ethical analysis has two parts: assembling a reliable and comprehensive account of the facts of the matter, drawing on available evidence in the descriptive medical ethics and other empirical literature; and identifying and clarifying concepts relevant to evaluating the ethical implications of this information. Argument-based ethical reasoning must be grounded in clinical reality if it aims to have clinical application and should use concepts that are clearly articulated.

Arguments organize these concepts into an argument: a coherent set of reasons that together support a conclusion for how one should or should not act. Reasons in arguments are expressed in terms of appeals to one or more general ethical frameworks.

DeGrazia and Beauchamp have recently identified and critically assessed five basic appeals.[2] The first appeal is to tradition and practice standards, the quality of which is a function of the ethical analysis and argument that support traditional beliefs and current practice standards. The second is to ethical principles such as respect for autonomy, beneficence, nonmaleficence, and justice.[3] When these principles are "specified," i.e. clarified in their relationship to clinical reality, they provide compelling action guides, as we have explained in previous chapters. The third is general ethical theory, of which there are two types predominant in the argument-based medical ethics literature: consequentialism (the justification of a course of action depends on whether consequences of the right sort result from it) and deontological approaches (the justification of a course of action is grounded in considerations other than consequences). The fourth is casuistry, which involves appeal to relevantly similar cases and applying the reasoning about these paradigm cases to the case at hand. The fifth is to what is called "reflective equilibrium," i.e. starting with considered judgments (those most likely to be free of bias) and exploring their joint implications for the principles that should together guide decision making and behavior. We would add a sixth, virtue-based appeals. These appeal to traits of character that physicians should cultivate as fiduciary professionals responsible for the care of patients and the management of health care organizations.

Some appeals are not acceptable in argument-based ethics. Sulmasy and Sugarman provide a useful account of these mistaken forms of reasoning in argument-based ethics.[4] First, historical practices do not by themselves justify conclusions. That something has been done or not done in the past, e.g. induced abortion, even if commonly done or prohibited, does not, by itself, justify our continuing to do or to prohibit it now. Second, majority opinions do not entail argument-based opinions, including majority opinions reported in well-designed surveys. The results of such studies provide important starting points for ethical analysis and argument but are no substitute for them. Third, the fact that something is permitted by law does not make it ethically permissible. The law is an important starting point for ethical analysis and argument, but should not be taken uncritically as the final word. The abortion controversy amply illustrates this point. Fourth, the opinions of experts do not in and of themselves count as the conclusions of well-reasoned arguments. Argument-based ethics papers and books should not be judged solely on the basis of their source – an individual physician, a research group, or a professional association – no matter how prominent and accomplished.[5] Instead, these works should be held to standards of intellectual rigor that are in their own way as demanding as those of evidence-based medicine and other standards for evaluating the medical and scientific literature. Fifth, the fact that something is biologically true does not by itself establish well-reasoned conclusions. It is an error to think that ethics can simply be derived from human biology.

Finally, it is often said that there is no right or wrong answer in ethics. This is a disservice to physicians turning to the argument-based medical ethics literature. There are well argued and poorly argued positions and they can be reliably distinguished. The latter appeal to "gut feeling," free-floating intuition, and unsystematic clinical ethical judgment and decision making, rather than judgment and decision making that meet standards of careful reflection and argument that are the hallmarks of argument-based medical ethics. Much of the current pro-life versus pro-choice public discourse about the ethics and public policy of abortion suffers from this shortcoming. The literature of perinatal ethics continues to grow, making it highly unlikely that there is no prior relevant literature that needs to be considered. Relevant literature should be cited and analyses and arguments from this literature should be presented clearly and accurately. In the basic and clinical science literature, investigators are increasingly expected to elucidate the search strategies, including key words, databases, bibliographies, and other sources used. This same standard should begin to be met by the argument-based ethics literature.

In preventing readers' bias, it is helpful to identify the disciplines represented among the authors. The argument-based medical ethics literature is distinctive in that work of high quality by non-clinicians should influence the clinical judgment and decision making of physicians, just as work on infectious diseases of the reproductive tract by microbiologists or on pharmacokinetics of gynecologic cancer chemotherapy by pharmacologists rightly influences clinical judgment and practice. Argument-based ethics scholarship, therefore, should not be dismissed when only some or even none of the authors are physicians.

At the same time, the reader should be aware of positive or negative bias toward an argument, based on the reputation of the author(s) or of the journal. Just as in the basic and clinical sciences, the standing of authors and journals in obstetrics and gynecology or in the field of bioethics is no guarantee of quality in argument-based medical ethics.

10.2.3 Step 3: What are the results of the argument?

The results of argument-based ethics are the conclusions of ethical analysis and argument. As emphasized above, they should be clearly stated and easy to find in the argument.

10.2.4 Step 4: How should I apply the results in clinical practice, research, or advocacy?

The results of argument-based medical ethics can be helpful in at least three ways. First, they may have important practical implications, especially if the results incorporate evidence to support the clinical utility of acting on the conclusions of an argument. Second, they may have important theoretical implications, which do not depend on whether an intervention was performed and evaluated. Identifying such theoretical implications results in critical assessment and revision of ethical frameworks and appeals based on them. Finally, readers of the perinatal ethics literature should ask themselves how they should change their thinking (clinical judgment and reasoning), attitudes (toward patients, their families, and legal institutions), clinical practice, research, or advocacy. This is a crucial step in the method of evidence-based reasoning, and therefore in the methods of argument-based ethics, because the fourth step relates directly to improving the quality of patient care, teaching, research, and organizational culture.

10.3 Conclusion

In this chapter, we have provided a tool based on the professional responsibility model of perinatal ethics that can be used to critically evaluate the literature of perinatal ethics.

10.4 References

1. McCullough LB, Coverdale JH, Chervenak FA. Argument-based medical ethics: a formal tool for critically appraising the normative medical ethics literature. Am J Obstet Gynecol 2004;191:1097–1102.
2. Degrazia D, Veauchamp TL. Philosophy: ethical principles and common morality. In Sugarman J, Sulmasy DP, eds. Methods in Medical Ethics, 2nd ed. Washington, DC: Georgetown University Press, 2010:37–53.
3. Bauchamp TL, Children JF. Principles of Biomedical Ethics, 7th ed. New York: Oxford University Press, 2012.
4. Sulmasy DP, Sugarman J. The many methods of medical ethics (or, thirteen ways of looking at a blackbird. In Sugarman J, Sulmasy DP, eds. Methods in Medical Ethics, 2nd ed. Washington, DC: Georgetown University Press, 2010:3–19.
5. Pellegrino ED. Codes, virtues, and professionalism. In Sugarman J, Sulmasy DP, eds. Methods in Medical Ethics, 2nd ed. Washington, DC: Georgetown University Press, 2010:91–107.

10.5 Summary points

- The literature of perinatal ethics should be critically appraised.
- A four-step tool that mirrors the process of critical appraisal of the scientific and clinical literature of perinatology equips the perinatologist to critically appraise the perinatal ethics literature.

11 Acknowledgements

The chapters of this book are in part adapted and include text from previously published work, used with permission.

Chapter 1

Chervenak FA, McCullough LB, Brent RL. The professional responsibility model of obstetric ethics: avoiding the perils of clashing rights. Am J Obstet Gynecol 2011;205:315.e1–5.
Chervenak FA, McCullough LB. Clinical guides to preventing ethical conflicts between pregnant women and their physicians. Am J Obstet Gynecol 1990;162:303–307.

Chapter 2

Chervenak FA, McCullough LB. An ethically justified, practical approach to offering, recommending, performing, and referring for induced abortion and infanticide. Am J Obstet Gynecol 2009;201:560.e1–6.

Chapter 3

Chervenak FA, McCullough LB. The limits of viability. J Perinat Med 1997;25:418–420.
Chervenak FA, McCullough LB, Levene MI. An ethically justified, clinically comprehensive approach to peri-viability: gynaecologic, obstetric, perinatal, and neonatal dimensions. J Obstet Gynaecol 2007;27:3–7.

Chapter 4

Chervenak FA, McCullough LB. An ethically justified algorithm for offering, recommending, and performing cesarean delivery and its application in managed care practice. Obstet Gynecol 1995;87:302–305.
Kalish RB, McCullough LB, Chervenak FA. Decision-making about caesarean delivery. Lancet 2006;367:883–45.
Chasen S, Chervenak FA, McCullough LB. The role of cephalocentesis in modern obstetrics. Am J Obstet Gynecol 2001;185:734–736.
Chervenak FA, McCullough LB. Non-aggressive obstetric management: an option for some fetal anomalies during the third trimester. JAMA 1989;261:3439–3440.
Chervenak FA, McCullough LB. Ethical dimensions of non-aggressive fetal management. Semin Fetal Neonatal Med 2008;13:316–319.

Chapter 5

Chervenak FA, McCullough LB, Brent RL, Levene LI, Arabin B. Planned home birth: the professional responsibility response. Am J Obstet Gynecol 2013;208:31–38.

Chervenak FA, McCullough LB, Grünebaum A, Arabin B, Levene MI, Brent RL. Planned home birth in the United States and professionalism: a critical assessment. J Clin Ethics 2013;24:184–191.

Chapter 6

McCullough LB, Coverdale JH, Chervenak FA. Ethical challenges of decision making with pregnant patients who have schizophrenia. Am J Obstet Gynecol 2002;187:696–702.

Chapter 7

Chervenak FA, McCullough LB, Arabin B. Why the Groningen Protocol should be rejected. Hastings Cent Rep 2006;36:30–33.

Chervenak FA, McCullough LB, Arabin B. The Groningen Protocol: Is it necessary? Is it scientific? Is it ethical? J Perinat Med 2009;37:199–205.

Chapter 8

Chervenak FA, McCullough LB. An ethically justified framework for clinical investigation to benefit pregnant and fetal patients. Am J Bioeth 2011;11:39–49.

Chapter 9

Chervenak FA, McCullough LB. Women and children first: transforming an historic defining moment into a contemporary ethical imperative. Am J Obstet Gynecol 2009;201:335.e1–5.

Chapter 10

McCullough LB, Coverdale JH, Chervenak FA. Argument-based medical ethics: a formal tool for critically appraising the normative medical ethics literature. Am J Obstet Gynecol 2004;191:1097–1102/

Index